RETHINKING LEARNING DISABILITIES

RETHINKING LEARNING DISABILITIES

Understanding Children Who Struggle in School

DEBORAH P. WABER

THE GUILFORD PRESS
New York London

© 2010 The Guilford Press
A Division of Guilford Publications, Inc.
72 Spring Street, New York, NY 10012
www.guilford.com

Paperback edition 2011

Printed in the United States of America

This book is printed on acid-free paper.

Last digit is print number: 9   8   7   6   5   4   3   2

Library of Congress Cataloging-in-Publication Data

Waber, Deborah P.
Rethinking learning disabilities : understanding children who struggle
in school / Deborah P. Waber.
    p. cm.
Includes bibliographical references and index.
ISBN 978-1-60623-565-2 (hardcover)
ISBN 978-1-4625-0334-6 (paperback)
  1. Learning disabled children—Education.   2. Learning disabilities.   I. Title.
LC4704.W3 2010
371.9—dc22

                                                           2009032138

About the Author

Deborah P. Waber, PhD, is Senior Associate in Psychology in the Department of Psychiatry at Children's Hospital Boston and Associate Professor of Psychology in the Department of Psychiatry at Harvard Medical School. Her research includes innovative work on the development of children with learning and attention disorders and large-scale studies of the typical development of schoolchildren. Dr. Waber has published peer-reviewed studies on related topics, including neuropsychological effects of therapy in childhood cancer patients and outcomes in children with neurogenetic disorders, prematurity, and early malnutrition. In addition to her research work, she has a clinical practice as Senior Neuropsychologist in the Learning Disabilities Program in the Department of Neurology at Children's Hospital Boston. She is also actively engaged in clinical training and mentoring young investigators.

Preface

In the mid-1960s educator Samuel Kirk introduced the term "learning disability" to describe children who struggled with their academic skills even though they had normal intellectual capacity. Prior to that time, it had too often been assumed that children who did poorly in school were simply slow learners, an assumption that would be significantly challenged by this new paradigm. Kirk's term, coming at the moment it did, helped to revolutionize the way that educators, physicians, and parents thought about and dealt with the many children who struggle in school. The term, and the thinking that motivated it, held that many normally intelligent children with school struggles had an intrinsic, neurologically based deficit that interfered with their ability to acquire a specific academic skill. This new paradigm came to be reflected in the scientific literature, in special education laws, in educational approaches, and more broadly in popular conceptions held by parents, teachers, and individuals with learning disabilities themselves. Use of the term "disability," importantly, put these learning problems on a par, both legally and clinically, with the category of motor and sensory disabilities. The disability itself, it was assumed, would be reliably and objectively identified by psychometrically rigorous tests, whose results could be evaluated against clear, empirically based criteria. For several decades this perspective seemed to work and to make good sense.

As the years went on, however, it became increasingly difficult to actually make the paradigm work in practice within the educational system. Despite volumes upon volumes of work, scholars are still unable to reach consensus about what a learning disability is, how to know if someone has it, and what to do about it. Equally important, as their consciousness has been raised about learning disabilities, parents' demand for services has grown dramatically, straining already scarce resources. As a result of all this, there are continual disputes about who "really" has a learning disability, and the system can be strained to the point of becoming dysfunctional. Too often, in response to these strains, the relationship between parents and schools deteriorates to an adversarial struggle, subverting the primary mission of the educational system itself—that is, to promote children's success in learning.

Despite the many problems that have arisen, however, the basic paradigm—the conceptual framework that shapes our understanding of children who struggle in school—has changed remarkably little in the half century since Kirk introduced the learning disability terminology. Yet given the growing dissatisfaction with the system, on all sides, the time is ripe for rethinking the whole enterprise. This rethinking must begin with the basic paradigm for understanding children who struggle.

This volume is based on the premise that learning disabilities are developmental in origin; that is, they are a manifestation of the lifelong processes of interaction between the child and environment. The phenomena captured by the term "learning disability" evolve as the child needs to adapt to the world that he or she must navigate. In order to succeed in school, children need not only to be able to efficiently decode words on a page or execute a math calculation accurately. They need to be able to accurately process and make meaning from the language they hear in classroom lectures or in conversations, to find the right words and assemble them into meaningful discourse to communicate their thoughts, to figure out what is important or not important to pay attention to, to accurately interpret social cues from adults or peers and to respond appropriately, to know when to abandon one problem-solving approach for another; the list is endless. Moreover, competencies do not develop as independent faculties, but in interaction with one another in the context of the developing child. Even though these phenomena are developmental in origin, however, the field of learning disabilities has only minimally attended to and integrated developmental theory.

Rethinking Learning Disabilities offers a different perspective, one that is firmly rooted in the broadest traditions of developmental science, especially developmental psychology and developmental cognitive neuroscience. It asserts that the concept of a "learning disability" is really about *the inherent incompatibility between normally occurring biological heterogeneity and socially determined expectations.* Within this developmental framework, the problem of children who struggle in school is not one of *disability* but rather one of *adaptation.* The proper focus of assessment, moreover, is thus not the skill or even the child, but rather the *interaction* between the child and the world within which that child must function.

The book provides a detailed theoretical argument, followed by case studies describing the clinical application of a developmental approach to real children. To be sure, a different perspective on learning disability will solve some problems and create others, but the current situation is fast becoming untenable. The term "learning disability" itself, which anchored the field for so long, continues to lose useful meaning. Moreover, as the system breaks down, valuable resources are diverted to struggles among parents, teachers, and administrators and thus away from the children whose needs they are meant to address.

For me, this book represents the logical culmination of a journey that began decades ago. While mastering the intricacies of Piaget's theory as a developmental psychology graduate student, I became convinced that a crucial element was missing from the prevailing approach to cognitive development: namely, the child's brain. It would be impossible, I believed, to truly know what motivates cognitive development without understanding its biology. My quest soon led me to what was at the time an infant field, neuropsychology, and its even newer subspecialty of developmental neuropsychology. Once exposed to what was for me an unbelievably fascinating and almost magical new neighborhood of psychological science, I was forever hooked.

My subsequent move into the learning disability world seemed serendipitous at the time, but in retrospect made perfect sense. I had been working in developmental neuropsychology research at Children's Hospital Boston for some years when I decided, with collegial supervision, to try my hand at clinical work. Learning disabilities particularly intrigued me, probably because of their presumed developmental origins and relatively subtle manifestations, which felt familiar given my background in developmental psychology. Thus, when offered an opportunity in the mid-1980s to join in the Learning Disabilities Program at Children's Hospital Boston, I seized it eagerly.

Because my intellectual roots, and thus my frame of reference, were not in clinical psychology but in developmental psychology, I viewed the problems encountered by children with learning problems not through the lens of pathology but through one of normal development. My developmental perspective, therefore, has taken me in a different direction from some others in the field, as I reference the problem to the developing system, in its broadest sense, rather than to deficits or symptoms. Although there are certainly similarities across children with school difficulties, for me each child is unique, because for each child this system is unique. To this day, every child I meet presents a new and intriguing problem to be solved, and every one stimulates evolution of my thinking.

The footprints of this journey can be found throughout the book. While writing it, I was surprised to find that seemingly diverse and unconnected pieces of knowledge from my past resurfaced and felt highly relevant. More important, they began to fit together in new and different ways. Piagetian theory, for example, turned out to be far more relevant to understanding learning disabilities than I had previously recognized, much less articulated to myself (Chapter 2), as was the comparative psychology of animal behavior (Chapter 3), which has always fascinated me. I also needed to learn a great deal that I had not known before, as I encountered new areas about which I knew less but whose importance became clear. For example, with the developmental perspective of the child in context, I realized that I needed a better understanding of the history of childhood in the United States to make sense of the learning disability concept (Chapter 2). Again, it was unexpected that this history would become so relevant to understanding children who struggle in school in the present day.

More than anything, however, both the book and I are the product of my own developmental context, especially the colleagues with whom I have been so fortunate to work through the years. I came to Children's Hospital Boston in 1974 to work with Peter Wolff, a brilliant and refreshingly iconoclastic child psychiatrist who remarkably shared many of my interests at the time. In addition to mentoring my career, he taught me the essential value of skepticism about the "accepted wisdom," uncomfortable though it may be, and reinforced my nascent inclinations in that direction. Peter was always right, however, and often maddeningly so. Through Peter, I met the incomparable Edith Kaplan, whose process approach to neuropsychology shaped my powers of clinical observation and understanding of the assessment process and of development. Edith, trained by Heinz Werner, was a different kind of neuropsychologist, and she passed the Wernerian developmental tradition down to her students. Peter also introduced me to Martha Denckla, a pioneer in pediatric behavioral neurology and then Director of the Learning Disabilities Program, whose wisdom and clarity of insight never cease to amaze me and who remains a touchstone for me to this day. It was through Edith that I met Jane Holmes Bernstein, who became a lifelong friend and colleague and always a teacher to me, as well as to countless trainees and other professionals throughout the world. Jane, a developmentalist with a vengeance and a voracious consumer of knowledge from remarkably diverse sources, pioneered the clinical application of neuropsychology to children. I have learned more from her than I probably know. She and I disagree about who coined the "child–world" system terminology, but I am quite convinced that the credit belongs to her.

My colleagues in the Learning Disabilities Program have also been my valued teachers over the past several decades, and in writing this book I stand on their capable shoulders. I consider myself forever fortunate to have joined that family. I look forward each week to our clinic meeting, knowing that my day will be stimulating and usually satisfying as we struggle together to make sense of each child in context. David Urion, the current director of the program, has taught me volumes with his encyclopedic knowledge not only of pediatric neurology and behavioral neurology (as well as other esoterica), but also of virtually every child whom we have ever seen.

From Grant Cioffi, Professor of Education and reading scholar, I learned the importance of assessing reading and writing in ecologically valid ways that provide a detailed understanding about how children solve the real-world challenge of deriving meaning from text and expressing their thoughts in the written word. His untimely death has been a profound loss, personally and professionally, to us all. Kristine Strand, Professor of Speech and Language Pathology, has taught me how to listen to children's language, how to describe it, and how to make sense of its impact on their lives. Grant and Kristine have helped me to understand the intimate and inseparable relationship between oral and written language, too often lost in the fractured world of disciplines.

Maria Marolda has provided endless insight into the multifaceted nature of children's mathematical learning and competencies—not just what they do, but how they do it and where the matches and mismatches with the curriculum occur. Together we have explored the remarkable symmetries to be found in mathematics learning and neuropsychology. I am grateful for her wisdom, her generous spirit, and her reliable common sense.

Finally, Bill Mitchell, an infinitely compassionate and sensible psychologist, has taught me about the behavioral and emotional manifestations and consequences of the "struggle" and their developmental course. His insight into the "mutually exacerbating" dynamic of cognition and affect in children who struggle in school is foundational in my understanding.

As David Urion once remarked, the learning disabilities team functions like the old Boston Celtics: Everyone knows where everyone else is on the court and what they are doing without the need to glance over their shoulder; everyone knows exactly where the ball is and will generously pass it. It is my honor and privilege to have had the opportunity to work with these talented experts in the program over the years. I am also enormously grateful to them for allowing me to use material from their evaluations for the case studies in the book.

I must also acknowledge the Department of Psychiatry at Children's Hospital Boston, especially William Beardslee, the former chair, and David DeMaso, the current chair, who have unfailingly supported my career through the years and generously given me the freedom to pursue my interests. My dear friend Larry Cohen endlessly encouraged me to write the book and cheered me on, teaching me the true meaning of the word *forward*. John and Eleanor Myers, likewise, offered welcome encouragement and thoughtful insights throughout the process. I am exceedingly grateful as well to my editors at The Guilford Press. Rochelle Serwator consistently provided gentle but firm and always wise advice, and Barbara Watkins's inspired editing brought the book to a whole new level.

Finally, I can never express in words my gratitude to my children, Abigail and Samuel Leonard, who generously and willingly shared their mother with her work at Children's Hospital while they were growing up—not easy for them, I know—and whose unflagging enthusiasm for this project has been a continuing source of joy for me.

Contents

PART I

THE DEVELOPMENTAL APPROACH TO LEARNING DISABILITIES

Chapter 1

The Dilemma

What Is a Learning Disability?

Thirty years of psychometric approaches have failed to
provide satisfactory answers to the learning disabilities
dilemma.
—CHRISTENSEN (1992)

Ten years later, little new research has been completed that
diminishes the veracity of this conclusion.
—FRANCES ET AL. (2005)

What is a learning disability and how do you know if a child has
it? This deceptively simple question has perplexed educators, researchers,
clinicians, and parents for decades. Questions about the possibility of a
learning disability can arise at any point in a child's school career when
a parent or teacher senses that something is "not right" about a child's
learning. For some children problems become apparent in preschool, for
some in kindergarten or first grade, and for still others, perhaps not
until middle or even high school. When parents request an evaluation,
they typically seek answers to two basic questions: "Does my child have
a learning disability?" and, if so, "What should be done about it?" On
the face of it, the first of these questions should be the easier of the two.
In fact, that is not necessarily the case. Although the term "learning disability" is widely used and accepted as a diagnosis by professionals and
laypeople, its definition has been remarkably elusive. The label has actually become less, rather than more, meaningful over time.

Two decades ago I wrote that "although most practitioners feel
fairly comfortable identifying a learning disabled child as such ... the
diagnosis is remarkably resistant to definition" (Waber, 1989, p. 29).

Since then, after much intensive research and debate, the situation has only grown more confusing. Experts continue to struggle to reach consensus about a diagnosis that is thought to afflict upward of 5% of all U.S. schoolchildren and is by far the fastest growing disability category in the public education system. This is a troubling state of affairs for a field that has benefited from substantial resources as well as the attention of many thoughtful experts for so many years. The struggle over the definition, however, is only a symptom of the far more fundamental confusion about the phenomenon itself.

An evaluation may fail to identify special needs using one set of tests whereas a different result is obtained with a different set of tests or even the same tests in another pair of hands. Or the test scores may fail to document a problem, while the child continues to struggle and becomes increasingly discouraged. The confusion only intensifies when the question arises as to "what kind of learning disability" the child has. One evaluator may diagnose attention-deficit/hyperactivity disorder (ADHD), whereas another concludes that there is a problem with "processing." Children may be labeled as visual or auditory learners, dysgraphic or dyslexic. Diagnoses such as "nonverbal learning disability" and more recently "executive function disorder" have arisen, as if to fill the endless need for more and more diagnostic labels because of the inadequacy of existing terminology to capture the diverse phenomenology of the children for whom these questions are raised.

The plight of children who come from economically disadvantaged communities and have learning problems is even more troubling. For them the diagnostic process can be far more difficult to navigate and the resources scarcer. A child who might be eligible for special education services in a suburban school system can languish in a depressed urban or rural community because of the overwhelming need, limited resources, or the absence of a savvy advocate. Such children are more likely to become discouraged and drop out of school, at great economic cost not only to themselves and their families but to the larger society, which is deprived of human potential. Other children with more complex cognitive, emotional, or behavioral problems may earn a learning disability designation because no other appropriate placement is available.

This confusion is also manifest in the periodically shifting diagnostic criteria. For many years, in most states, a child needed to exhibit a severe discrepancy between ability and achievement to qualify for special education services under the learning disability category, with specific criteria determined on a state-by-state basis because regulations were promulgated at the state level. Since the discrepancy criterion is now acknowledged to be flawed (Francis et al., 2005), the most recent revision of the federal law states that it can no longer be used to deprive a child of needed services. It is no wonder that parents, teachers, and administrators become frustrated and bewildered as they strive to remain in compliance with the law and manage shrinking resources while meeting children's rights to a "free and appropriate public education."

Nonetheless, the need for some rational and effective strategy to deal with the many children, who, everyone agrees, have a "problem" is incontrovertible. If not addressed adequately, the impact of these problems can snowball, affecting multiple aspects of children's development in functionally significant ways. Repeated and unacknowledged experiences of failure and frustration can lead to disengagement from the academic process, with further psychosocial and adaptive fallout.

When a child appears to struggle, it is reasonable to consider the possibility of a learning disability, but the response to this consideration is by no means simple or straightforward. Often, the prevailing legal definitions and research-based criteria are difficult to reconcile with the more complex picture that parents and teachers observe on a daily basis. When the system works well, the problem is identified, the appropriate educational services are implemented, and the child makes academic progress. Sometimes, however, things do not go so well. Parents may struggle to understand whether their child does or does not fit the descriptions they read about or hear from experts, advocacy groups, or websites, and teachers may become frustrated when problems persist despite their attempts to apply what they believe to be good practices. For them, as well as parents, the process is often one of trial and error, as they try to figure out "what's going on" with the child and shift approaches to fit their various theories (e.g., lack of investment, ADHD, dyslexia). Children, meanwhile, can become discouraged as their self-efficacy is eroded, with significant consequences for their psychosocial adjustment. School systems may deny needed services because of resource limitations or philosophical differences, while parents may harbor unrealistic expectations of what a school can reasonably provide or accomplish, even with appropriate supports in place.

THE GAP BETWEEN POLICY AND PRACTICE

The all-too-frequent gap between the formal, legally defined systems and the actual experience of children, families, educators, and clinicians reflects the fact that policy has very different goals from clinical practice. The primary goal of policy is to differentiate children who do or do not qualify legally for an entitlement in order to triage finite resources;

the primary goal of clinical practice is to describe the individual child's developmental needs and determine how they can best be met.

In order to achieve the policy goal, the diagnostic process needs to consist of relatively simple and empirically specifiable and replicable standards that can be directly referenced to legal regulations. This goal is difficult to achieve if one retains a clinical focus on the complexities of an individual developing child. The job becomes easier, however, if the focus is restricted to specific academic skills that can be easily and reliably measured. Often, however, these discrete skills may constitute only one element of the clinical picture. Furthermore, because the law applies to children with "disabilities," physical and cognitive alike, the learning disability diagnosis, which is in reality dimensional, needs to be defined categorically, like the physical disabilities, a process that will inevitably be forced. The characterization of the learning disability diagnosis in the research and policy worlds is often at variance with actual situations encountered "on the ground." Users of the special education system, therefore, are often left feeling baffled, unsatisfied, frustrated, or angry, as they struggle to understand how a particular child does or does not "qualify."

Although the legal system is internally rational, it promotes an unfortunate conceptualization of the child as a product. This "industrial" model is valid in the policy arena as a practical means to allocate limited resources, but it can be less helpful to parents, teachers, and ultimately to the children whose development they seek to facilitate.

WIDE VARIATION AMONG CHILDREN WITH LEARNING PROBLEMS

To complicate matters, children who have trouble with specific academic skills, such as reading or mathematics, more often than not exhibit difficulties in other cognitive realms that can themselves affect school success, both academically and socially (Morris et al., 1998; Waber, Forbes, Wolff, & Weiler, 2004). Moreover, many children can master the fundamentals of reading and calculation and do not have a primary disorder of attention, yet they struggle in school. They may not qualify for official recognition, and their success can depend on the sensitivity and skills of a particular teacher, the advocacy and support of a parent, or private tutoring arrangements. Evidence-based approaches to skill development (i.e., those with efficacy demonstrated in controlled clinical trials) can provide a *necessary* instructional component for many children; often, however, they are not *sufficient* to meet their individual needs as they develop. There is growing recognition that some children are "repaired" by evidence-based interventions in the early years—learning to decode words based on phonologically based interventions—only to have problems surface later on, in related or seemingly unrelated arenas. Some children may experience problems that become florid one year but are well managed the next, largely because of the classroom environment and the insight (or lack of insight) of a particular teacher. In short, there is enormous individual variation among children with learning problems—a fact that is not transparent from much of the research literature because it focuses so narrowly on specific skills.

Research in learning disabilities has been increasingly motivated by, and tied to, these policy considerations; the tail may be wagging the dog. As a result, the research has focused more and more narrowly on discrete skills—reading, writing, and calculation—and even on specific components of these skills. Fundamental to this perspective is the premise that the functional origin of the problem as well as the child's other characteristics and circumstances are irrelevant. The preferred strategy is to identify the skill deficit, focus on it, and then repair it as a project in cognitive engineering. The appeal of such an approach is its rationality and internal consistency; discrete skills can be reliably measured, with exquisite psychometric precision, for purposes of both identification and intervention. The ultimate goal of this research is to demonstrate empirically, using randomized trial methodology adopted from clinical medicine, that the outcomes, measured in terms of skill levels, are superior in the experimental arm of the study relative to the control arm, thus providing data to support "evidence-based" practice. This approach is eminently rational. If the child meets specified psychometrically defined criteria for a reading or math disability, he or she is given a diagnosis of specific learning disability, and the school then defines specific goals and provides services using good evidence-based practices accordingly, parallel to the physical disabilities.

In the real world, however, the observations that trigger a question of a learning disability are anything but straightforward:

- "My child has been receiving some reading help since first grade; his reading has improved a lot, but now homework is becoming a battle. *Does he have a learning disability?*"
- "The kindergarten teacher thought my child was not mature enough for first grade, so we held her back, but now that she's in first grade, she's still struggling to get her seatwork done. She prefers to socialize in class and she's starting to have stomachaches in the morning. *Does she have a learning disability?*"
- "My child typically starts off the year OK but then the grades start to fall off by Thanksgiving. Each year it seems to be getting worse. *Does he have a learning disability?*"

- "My child learned to read without too much trouble in first grade, but now in the fourth grade she's having more trouble getting her work done, and she seems to have trouble keeping friends. *Does she have a learning disability?*"
- "A child in my class comes from a bilingual home, and her single mother, who speaks little English, works at night while the teen-age sister takes care of her. She's hardworking but just can't seem to keep up. *Does she have a learning disability?*"
- "My child has always had to work hard, but his grades have been fine. Now he gets upset and at times belligerent when he has a writing assignment. *Is he just lazy or does he have a learning disability?*"
- "My child seems to know what she's doing when we go over the work at home, but she does poorly on the tests when she is in school. *Does she have a learning disability?*"

Answering this apparently simple question is no easy feat. Of course, one can resort to a decision rule based on fundamental psychometric measurement criteria, but how well can such an approach actually mitigate these children's problems?

As research and policy become ever more skill-focused, parents and teachers continue to grapple with developing human beings. They view the skill deficits as the cardinal symptom of the problem, yet they also recognize the complex and developmentally dynamic cognitive and social processes that more often than not accompany the specific skill problem. These processes can have a functional impact on academic and psychosocial well-being that is as great, or sometimes greater, than the skill deficit itself. Parents and teachers may restrict their focus to the skill problem, assuming that other potentially relevant aspects of the child's functioning are ineligible for consideration. There is no simple and reliable empirical test to measure these other characteristics, nor is there a sanctioned label to apply. Often they try to understand the multiple and heterogeneous accompanying issues as a symptom of the child's "dyslexia" or "ADHD" because they have no other accepted way to understand them.

THE LIMITATIONS OF PSYCHOEDUCATIONAL TESTS

Another problem is the psychoeducational tests themselves. Many of the widely used psychoeducational tests employ short discrete items rather than the lengthier and more complex material that is ecologically representative of curricular demands. Test construction is necessarily oriented to psychometric criteria, which can be difficult to achieve in more complex and ecologically relevant materials. Many times, children do not qualify for special consideration because they have grade-level performance (as measured by psychoeducational tests), even though they are plainly in trouble on a day-to-day basis in their classrooms. Some of these children struggle and become discouraged, unless they happen to encounter a perceptive teacher who is willing to look beyond documented "normal" scores on psychoeducational testing.

One premise about which there is little disagreement, however, is that the phenomena associated with the learning disability construct, whatever they may be, are *neurodevelopmental in origin.* Curiously, the prevailing skill-based paradigms for understanding these problems are not actually developmental. Of course, researchers and educators attend carefully to the linear evolution of literacy and math skills across age and grade levels. Yet paying attention to age and linear progressions is not equivalent to paying attention to development. A developmental approach requires that the phenomena of interest—in this case, school problems—be seen within the broader theoretical context of developmental science, including developmental psychology and developmental cognitive neuroscience. This perspective, which has been largely missing from the discussion, can arguably point to a way out of the "learning disabilities dilemma."

ABOUT THIS BOOK

This book outlines an *explicitly developmental strategy* for solving the learning disabilities dilemma. This approach by no means detracts from the merit of well-researched approaches to remediate particular skills. Rather, it argues that these approaches are necessary but not sufficient to solve the problem. It thus *complements* more skill-focused approaches by furnishing a principled framework for their application within the context of the developing child. For teachers, administrators, and even policymakers, it can provide a rationale for organizing and managing these difficult and complex questions. Most important, it shifts the focus of effort from the often contentious and capricious process of eligibility decisions about who does or does not have a "specific learning disability" to a project of informed and collaborative problem solving for children.

The balance of this chapter takes a closer look at problems with the way learning disabilities are currently understood and at attempts to solve those problems. Chapters 2 through 6 then present a developmental perspective on learning disabilities, starting with core principles

(Chapter 2) and key findings from developmental science (Chapter 3). Learning disabilities are developmental problems, and development is systemic in nature. As the research in Chapter 4 indicates, a lifespan perspective is fundamental when approaching a child with learning problems. There may be early predictors in infancy, and a developmental perspective is also essential to maximizing long-term outcomes when learning-disabled children grow up. In Chapters 5 and 6 I return to the issue of identification with insights from research conducted by myself and colleagues at Children's Hospital Boston as well as from contemporary cognitive neuroscience research. Part II of this book presents case studies that illustrate, in concrete terms, a strategy for putting the developmental framework described in Part I into practice.

"SPECIFIC LEARNING DISABILITY" AS A LEGAL CONSTRUCT

The term "learning disability" was first used in 1963 by the educator Samuel Kirk at a conference convened in Chicago by a group of parents whose children had what were referred to at that time as "perceptual handicaps" that impaired their school functioning. Too often, they believed, their children were misunderstood by schools, who dismissed them as cognitively deficient (Kirk, 1963; Shepherd, 2001).

Kirk used the term to refer to a group of children who harbored a neurologically based deficit in the acquisition of specific academic skills but whose mental development was not globally impaired. The term "learning disability" captured the spirit of their concerns. Specifically, these children were not globally low functioning; rather, they were individuals with normal intellectual capacity with a separable, but hidden, neurological *disability* that affected their learning, analogous to sensory or motor disabilities. This meeting led to the founding of the Association for Children with Learning Disabilities (ACLD), later to become the Learning Disabilities Association of America (LDA), a leading advocacy group.

Kirk's use of the word *disability* proved to be a brilliant stroke for advocacy, rapidly achieving translation into policy, in part because of a groundswell of support from advocates and in part because of the country's focus on civil rights in the 1960s. The term deftly captured the notion that the affected children were of normal intellect and attributed the school failure to a specific and circumscribed neurological defect or disability, comparable in status to other disability conditions. The first national legislation pertaining to learning-disabled children was passed 6 years later. The Children with Specific Learning Disabilities Act of

1969 was the first law passed by Congress to provide federal funding for education and research for the children to whom that label was applied (Shepherd, 2001). In that law, the term "specific learning disability" was first given official status, as follows:

> The term "children with specific learning disabilities" means those children who have a disorder in one or more of the basic psychological processes involved in understanding or in using language, spoken or written, which disorder may manifest itself in imperfect ability to listen, think, speak, read, write, spell or do mathematical calculations. Such disorders include such conditions as perceptual handicaps, brain injury, minimal brain dysfunction, dyslexia and developmental aphasia. Such [a] term does not include children who have learning problems which are primarily the result of visual, hearing, or motor handicaps, of mental retardation, of emotional disturbance, or of environmental disadvantage. (Public Law No. 91-230, 84 Stat., pp. 175, 177)

Learning disabilities would not be recognized legally as a disability category until 1975. However, the original 1969 definition has endured for decades, essentially unchanged even in the most recent reauthorization of the Individuals with Disabilities Education Act (IDEA), which, as we shall see, introduced radical changes in the identification process.

The law's language requires that the phenomenology be defined as a *disability* in order to make the case for much needed attention and publicly financed resources. Since the science needed to be aligned with the advocacy, and hence the policy, the law's language would set the course for the research and theory that was to follow. Moreover, the advocacy raised consciousness among parents and educators. As a result, the question of a learning disability was raised for more and more children with heterogeneous needs who were encountering legitimate school difficulties, many of whom did not fit the conceptualizations of the original advocates. Since the entitlements conferred by this legislation were associated with desirable resources, the identification process would become increasingly contentious as more and more parents became aware of their children's potential rights and came forward to request, and sometimes demand, resources for their children.

INTERPRETING THE LAW IN THE SCHOOLS

The number of children identified as learning disabled has skyrocketed in a way that its early advocates never could have foreseen. The "specific learning disability" designation now accounts for over half the children served by special education services in the United States. Some critics have argued that this high rate indicates that we are overidentifying children with learning disabilities (Kavale & Forness, 2003), providing services for children who are not *truly* learning disabled. Even these commentators, however, have no formula for deciding who truly has a learning disability, hoping that such diagnostic criteria will emerge from the neuroscientific arena. But as I elaborate in Chapters 5 and 6, the notion that some incontrovertible biological marker exists to be discovered may itself be fallacious. It is just as likely that the escalating identification rate is a legitimate symptom that schooling, as currently organized, is not appropriately equipped to effectively educate the broad range of children with diverse educational and social needs in accordance with the social demands of an increasingly information-based economy.

For many years the *specific learning disability* designation required that psychometric testing demonstrate a statistically significant *discrepancy* between ability and achievement, capturing in empirical terms the core concept. In many states the exact magnitude of the qualifying discrepancy was specified. This strategy was predicated on the basic concept that a learning disability involves unexpected school failure in the context of normal intelligence and adequate instruction. Inherent in this concept is the assumption that a "specific" learning disability involves a *modular*—that is, discrete and encapsulated—academic skill deficit in the context of otherwise normal functioning. This specific deficit, it follows, can be appropriately understood and therefore remediated without regard to the broader cognitive and social developmental context.

In reality, schools are frequently swayed when making placement decisions by considerations other than whether a child meets a strict legal or research-guided "definition." What a child needs to succeed in a particular setting or what resources are actually available are often just as important. This substantial gap in real life between standard definitions for identification and actual school practices in eligibility determinations, long observed by practitioners, is well documented empirically (Bocian, Beebe, MacMillan, & Gresham, 1999; Gresham, MacMillan, & Bocian, 1998; Kavale & Reese, 1992; MacMillan, Gresham, & Bocian, 1998). MacMillan and colleagues (1998) reported that although only 30% of the children referred for evaluation in their study met psychometric criteria for a specific learning disability, 54% were actually identified as such by school assessment teams. These decisions were not capricious (Bocian et al., 1999). Teachers and schools appeared to factor actual classroom achievement and behavior into their decisions, in addition to formal test scores, and they considered other contextual factors such as the normative performance of children at the local level, program availability, and the relative skills of particular teachers.

In addition, practitioners have sometimes turned to Section 504 legislation to meet the legitimate needs of children whose psychometric testing does not result in a designation of a specific learning disability. This legislation guarantees civil rights to people with disabilities and is legally in the purview of general education, not special education. A "504 plan" is frequently invoked to provide accommodations when it is apparent that something more needs to be done, but the child did not qualify for special education. Simply calling attention to the child's cognitive profile can sometimes have the salutary effect of relieving the child from an attribution of "moral turpitude" and stimulating teachers to entertain more positive and supportive attitudes. Thus, these categories and legal designations are far more fluid in practice than they appear on paper, as various players devise strategies to adjust the "fit" for children who are struggling academically while still meeting legal prescriptions.

In the end, educators are pragmatists; they navigate the existing institutional and legal structures to achieve goals that make sense, given the various constraints and resources available to them. Their behavior is an adaptive use of a system to meet genuine need in whatever way it can within the existing constraints. Bocian and colleagues (1999) commented that "teachers may be 'imperfect tests' but in terms of classroom relevance, their perceptions outrank student performance on isolated tasks in ideal, pristine conditions" (p. 12). A corollary to this observation is that research that is based on formally recognized identification criteria, whatever they may be, will have limited application to the challenges of the typical day-to-day life of schoolchildren, teachers, and administrators.

From a parent's perspective, concerns often center not only on skill development, but also on risks for discouragement, frustration, and eroding self-esteem, regardless of whether test scores confirm the specific learning disability designation. Teachers are typically not privy to the extent of the psychological fallout when children struggle on a daily basis with frustration, confusion, and helplessness. Parents, on the other hand, may face "meltdowns" at home in a child who appears well adjusted and compliant all day in class. For parents who are attuned to their children's moods and attitudes, this dynamic can cause considerable distress. The mounting concerns of parents, who understandably feel compelled to advocate for their child, can lead to pitched battles with school administrators, who are often responding to countervailing pressures to conserve limited economic resources and may ultimately be more focused on budgetary implications. School personnel look to test scores as a tool to provide a justifiable and fair basis for decisions. Everyone is caught in the turmoil, and no one is happy—especially the child who is the object of this attention. To help sort out the confusion, it is useful to step back and look at how these problems in identification developed.

EVOLUTION OF THE LEARNING DISABILITIES CONCEPT

In their account of the history of learning disabilities in the United States, Hallahan and Mock (2003) identify five distinct periods. The first four are fairly straightforward. According to them, the *European foundation period* (1800–1920) begins with the 19th-century neurologists who established the principles of localization of function and ends with reports of congenitally based conditions that mimic adult brain damage, such as Pringle-Morgan's (1896) first report of "congenital word blindness" and later Hinshelwood's (1917) book on the same topic. The *U.S. foundation period* (1920–1960) begins with compulsory education, the introduction of remedial programs into the schools, and the emergence of experts, such as Samuel Orton, who hypothesized that reading and learning problems stem from mixed hemispheric dominance, and Marianne Frostig, who focused on movement and visual perception. The *emergent period* (1960–1975) captures the transition from learning disability as a psychological construct to its recognition, in a series of legislative actions, as a disability on par with sensory and motor disabilities. The *solidification period* (1975–1985) began the focus on empirically valid research. This was a relatively calm period, during which schools began to implement the laws, and controversy was relatively limited.

Most interesting from our perspective is the final period, which Hallahan and Mock (2003) call the *turbulent period*. Although the dates they assign range from 1985 to 2000, the turbulence surely continues into the present. The IQ–achievement discrepancy definition (i.e., a statistically valid and reliable discrepancy between IQ and reading or math skill) had, for many years, been accepted fairly uncritically, because it intuitively captured the intent of Kirk's (1962) terminology. The noted British psychiatric epidemiologist, Sir Michael Rutter, moreover, had provided substantial data contrasting "backward readers" with those with "specific reading impairment," the latter characterized by a discrepancy between cognitive ability and reading skill that was absent in the former (Rutter & Yule, 1975). As the number of students identified as learning disabled continued to escalate, however, schools became entangled in sometimes contentious struggles with families, and researchers began to question assumptions. Issues that had been viewed as settled became controversial, escalating in intensity.

By the 1990s, the discrepancy definition itself had begun to attract greater scrutiny. Researchers critiqued the original Rutter and Yule analyses as methodologically flawed (Fletcher et al., 1994). Moreover, poor readers with and without a discrepancy were found to be indistinguishable in many ways, not only in terms of the reading itself but also in relation to associated language functions (Shaywitz, Fletcher, Holahan, & Shaywitz, 1992; Stanovich & Siegel, 1994). The epidemiological data indicated, however, that children who did meet criteria for a learning disability had higher IQs and, significant from a perspective of equity, better educated mothers (Shaywitz et al., 1992). Moreover, increasingly the discrepancy definition was invoked to exclude children rather than to include them and provide services.

As the discrepancy definition came under increasing attack, learning disability researchers redeployed their focus to specific academic skills, almost exclusively reading, and its cognitive underpinnings. Phonological processing, in particular, became the theoretical linchpin of much of the research in the 1990s, narrowing the focus from the child to the skill and then to a discrete cognitive component of the specific skill. As this highly modular approach gained currency, the concept of a developmental disorder receded. Although this strategy made the research task easier, the "learning disability" construct became increasingly muddled, and the theoretical basis from which to derive a consensual definition of learning disability was eroded. Equally significant, these children's other cognitive and affective issues came to be treated as troublesome "noise," rather than as functionally relevant, albeit heterogeneous, constituents of the child's problems (Morris et al., 1998; Stanovich & Siegel, 1994). As time went on, it became clear that the phonological processing deficiency was only one part of the reading problem. Intervention trials aimed at remediating this core cognitive deficit succeeded in improving word decoding and recognition, but were less successful at improving fluency and, importantly, comprehension, the ultimate goal of text reading.

As the learning disability diagnosis gained greater acceptance and more and more children presented the question of learning disability, the problem of "legitimate" need became more, rather than less, troubling. Ironically, while educational research provides an ever-growing armamentarium of potentially effective tools for working with children who have learning problems (Swanson, Harris, & Graham, 2003), the battleground remains the gatekeeper function. Schools and government entities have regarded with alarm the ever-growing numbers of students referred. Identification and referral remain a constant source of friction between families and schools.

Another significant development was the arrival of education reform in the form of the No Child Left Behind Act of 2001 (NCLB). NCLB was a response to concerns about the continued failure of U.S.

schools to educate all of their students appropriately, especially those from historically disadvantaged minority groups. The major innovation of NCLB was the institution of standards-based testing at nearly every grade level. According to the model, testing would identify failing students and schools, and measures would be taken to remediate their skill deficits. Thus, the strategy is one of quality control, similar to strategies that monitor product quality in industry. *Accountability* was the watchword of the legislation; if children were failing, someone was to be held accountable. Teachers and school administrators could be held accountable for children's failure to make progress, and children were themselves to be held responsible for their own achievement, eventually being denied a high school diploma if they failed to meet quality control standards.

It is within this historical, political, and social environment that the IDEA was reauthorized in 2005. Because the discrepancy definition had fallen into disfavor, there was the will to implement new strategies to effectively manage the ever-growing number of children being identified as learning disabled. Although the definition of a "specific learning disability" remained essentially unchanged in the 2005 reauthorization, the act introduced radically different provisions. Schools could continue to use the discrepancy definition to *include* children, but they could no longer *exclude* children from services if the discrepancy criterion was not met.

The legislation signaled the impending demise of the psychometric approach to identification. David Francis and his colleagues, over the years, have provided the most extensive and comprehensive body of research on psychometrically based strategies for learning disability identification. In 2005 they summarized the status of the field (Francis et al., 2005), presenting multiple analyses, complete with detailed scatterplots of thousands of student scores, that illustrated potential problems with psychometric definitions based on a single assessment. In their epidemiological database, over 30% of children identified as learning disabled by standard psychometric criteria (either low achievement and/or discrepancy) in the third grade no longer met the same criterion in the fifth grade. Quoting Christensen (1992), who wrote that "thirty years of psychometric approaches have failed to provide satisfactory answers to the learning disabilities dilemma" (p. 276), they commented that "ten years later, little new research has been completed that diminishes the veracity of this conclusion" (p. 106). They concluded that test scores should be a part of the decision-making progress, but that other behavioral considerations should be included as well. Measuring change over time, they argued, would be superior to the approach of capturing a single moment in time. How this strategy would be practically accomplished and what it would add remains a major question, however, because it continues to limit its scope to psychometrically driven test scores.

A NEW STRATEGY FOR IDENTIFICATION: RESPONSIVENESS TO INTERVENTION

Given the failure of the psychometric approaches to identification, experts have advocated a response-to-intervention (RTI) model (Fletcher, Francis, Morris, & Lyon, 2005; Fuchs & Fuchs, 2006), which is nonetheless psychometrically driven. This RTI model would encompass both evidence-based instruction and frequent testing of core skills to ferret out those children whose learning issues appeared intractable. Such children would represent "true" learning disability. In the 2005 reauthorization of the IDEA, states were given the alternative option of an RTI approach to identification, which has the added advantage of compatibility with NCLB. RTI models integrate programs of increasingly intensive instruction into the general education curriculum, focusing more attention on the "prereferral" process as a strategy to limit the number of learning disability referrals to those with genuine need (i.e., those who fail to respond to evidence-based instruction). At each level, children are assessed to identify those students who are inadequately responsive and who therefore require intervention at the next, more intensive, level in the system (Fuchs & Fuchs, 2006).

RTI is commanding attention as the most promising solution to the long-standing dilemma of identification. Moreover, it has the added benefit of prevention, since the RTI model enhances the prereferral, general education component of the process. There are two broad versions of this system. The *standard protocol model* (SPM), consistent with the spirit of the NCLB, focuses almost entirely on "evidence-based" instruction and rigorous testing. According to the most prevalent version of this system, all children must be given the benefit of scientifically validated, evidence-based instruction in the general education setting (called *Tier I*). Achievement is measured regularly, and those who fall behind are provided with more intensive group-based tutoring (*Tier II*). Those who are successful in such tutoring programs then return to the general education classroom. Those who fail to meet the goal at Tier II then become eligible for special education intervention.

The alternative *problem-solving model* (PSM) is less explicitly defined; it provides a conceptual framework but leaves the details to those who apply it. It too calls for levels of intensity and prereferral assessment, but the approaches to intervention are focused on problem solving at the individual level rather than a standardized curricular protocol. Curriculum-based measurement (CBM), targeted to curricular goals, can be used to identify children who are in academic trouble. Problem-solving teams act as consultants to the classroom teacher, and interventions address not just specific curricular approaches but the multiple issues that may be associated with the child's failure to make adequate progress.

The SPM, as it has been described and implemented in formal research, is distinctly modular in its provenance, whereas the PSM admits greater consideration of the whole child and more individualized strategies. Each predictably embodies strengths and weaknesses. The SPM is strong on reliability but lacks flexibility and provides no formal framework with which to consider the multiple developmental issues and contexts that impinge on individual children's school performance. The PSM approach, in contrast, is stronger on flexibility and the ability to accommodate these multiple considerations, but can be variable in its implementation and highly dependent on the skills and judgment of its practitioners. Evaluation of its effectiveness, moreover, can be a challenge, since the intervention can theoretically vary from child to child.

Most research-oriented proponents (Fuchs & Fuchs, 2006; VanDerHeyden, Witt, & Gilbertson, 2007) have clearly emphasized the SPM, in line with the overriding emphasis, among rigorous empirical researchers, on reliability and validity in assessment and on evidence-based clinical-trial approaches to intervention. Taken out of context, the SPM strategies make logical sense, much as NCLB has its own internal logic. It sets standards, identifies outliers—that is, those who fall outside the expected range—and then focuses on normalizing the performance of those outliers through clearly defined approaches with scientifically validated merit.

Yet, as with many apparently simple and straightforward ideas, the devil is in the details. For example, SPM is based on the predicate that children will be exposed to curricula that are proven scientifically to be effective, or evidence based. Although such curricula exist for early reading acquisition (and even then the proof of efficacy often does not extend to the more complex cognitive tasks of rate and comprehension), few programs are available for children who are no longer in that age group. Table 1.1 lists reading and math interventions reviewed on the website of the Institute of Educational Sciences "What Works Clearinghouse" (*ies.ed.gov/ncee/wwc*) as of September 2008. The limited availability of scientifically validated evidence-based programs is apparent. The vast majority of the programs reviewed pertain to beginning reading, and of these, only one (a program intended for first graders only) was

TABLE 1.1. Evidence-Based Efficacy Ratings of Elementary Reading and Mathematics Programs Based on Findings from the U.S. Department of Education Institute of Educational Sciences "What Works Clearinghouse"

	Total evaluable	Positive n (%)	Potentially positive n (%)	Mixed n (%)	No effect n (%)	Negative n (%)
Alphabetic	18	6 (33)	11 (61)	0	1 (9)	0
Fluency	11	0	7 (64)	0	4 (36)	0
Comprehension	19	0	7 (37)	2 (11)	7 (37)	2 (11)
General reading	5	1 (20)	4 (80)	0	0	0
Mathematics	5	0	1 (20)	0	4 (80)	0

Note. A total of 193 reading programs were listed, of which 23 were evaluable, and 74 mathematics programs, of which 5 were evaluable.

clearly effective. Thus, the availability of a sufficient armamentarium of evidence-based programs at the present time is problematic.

Also, SPM assumes that the prevention measures will set children on the right course and that benefits will accrue throughout their school careers. But what happens after the early primary grades? What if the goal is not simply being able to read a list of words but to comprehend and use text in a meaningful way, or to organize ideas and write about them? What if, as so often happens, the child who receives remediation in the early grades once again encounters difficulties in higher grades, in the remediated domain or some other? Another problem is the sheer volume of testing that needs to be done to track students and the very limited nature, therefore, of the assessment that is possible. One comprehensive multiyear systemwide test of such a model, for example, was based on 2-minute tests of basic fluency in oral word reading and computation (VanDerHeyden et al., 2007). It is unclear how well this remarkably narrow evaluation translated to academic function, especially if measured in terms of the real goals of learning after the early primary years.

As Mastropieri and Scruggs (2005) enumerate, the problems to be solved if the SPM is to work are potentially endless. How are general education teachers to be trained in the appropriate scientifically based curricula? Who monitors the general education teachers for treatment fidelity? What curricula are available for the K–12 range for all content areas? How will RTI be implemented at the middle and high school levels? Who has the ultimate authority to move students up or down? How will parents be involved in the process and what are their rights under this system? What about the student who meets criterion at Tier

II, returns to the classroom, and then begins to struggle again? How does SPM RTI deal with the multifaceted nature of problems in children with learning disorders? Do we envision multiple evidence-based curricula and multiple tiers operating simultaneously? The possibilities go on and on.

Moreover, as Mellard, Deshler, and Barth (2004) found when they convened focus groups of "street-level workers" and consumers, the technology or tool used, be it an RTI model or a discrepancy model, is only one component of a broader context that will always be equally, if not more, important. The informants confirmed that learning disability determination is, in large part, a function of the setting within which it is implemented. In general, they believed that resource availability typically had a greater influence on student identification than the extent to which the child met formal criteria for a disability. Instructional staff reported that they could much more readily justify why a student needed specialized instruction than whether the student actually had a learning disability. Parents also were less concerned about disability determination than the quality of the services that were actually received.

Second, and surprisingly, a number of participants were skeptical about the value of the specific learning disability category altogether. Many learning disability teachers, in particular, questioned its value, given the controversy it generates and the needs of a larger number of students within most schools than can be realistically categorized as learning disabled. Many educators felt that resources designated for children with learning disability should be made available to schools for addressing the needs of a broader number of students. Those charged with the task of assessment were generally more confident about their findings relative to the curricula in their school than to broader generic criteria for learning disability designation based on nationally standardized testing.

Third, many learning disability teachers complained that they were called upon to pitch in for so many tasks that they were unclear as to whether the specialized services students with learning disability needed were truly available. General education teachers were concerned about how they could handle the increasing pressures to teach to the state-required standards for content at the same time as they were being called upon to do specialized skill instruction and progress monitoring, as an RTI model might require. In general, nevertheless, these stakeholders believed that the ideal strategy for handling learning disabilities would be an efficient process that was somehow validated and tied to research, while also sensitive to age and developmental considerations.

The less rigorous PSM seems to have proven easier, if by no means easy, to actually implement than the more prominently featured SPM. The city of Minneapolis, for example, instituted such a program about a decade ago and has been fairly successful in systemwide implementation (Marston, Muyskens, Lau, & Canter, 2003). After obtaining a waiver from the state, they abandoned the categorical designation of learning disability in favor of a problem-solving RTI approach. There were three basic steps to the process: (1) Describe the student's problem with specificity, (2) generate and implement strategies for instructional intervention, and (3) monitor student progress and evaluate the effectiveness of the intervention. The school system instituted intervention assistance teams made up of professionals from within the building, including other teachers, who collaborated to develop and test solutions. The more intensive special education evaluations and placements were invoked if the problem-solving approach was not successful. As with other RTI efforts, the number of formal special education assessments decreased. There was also increased collaboration across the general education–special education boundaries. Contrary to what some had predicted, abandoning the learning disability designation in favor of the more open PSM for students in need did not open the floodgates. The number of students identified basically equaled the number of students who had formerly been identified with a learning disability. Indeed, approximately 75% of the students who had been identified by the PSM met the standard criteria for learning disability or mild-to-moderate mental impairment. In terms of skill levels, the performance of students identified by the learning disability and PSM strategies was very comparable. Another positive outcome was that the overidentification of minority students for special education that had existed prior to the introduction of RTI was normalized. Minority students were now identified in proportion to their numbers in the school system.

Thus, although there is no evidence that outcomes were superior in terms of actual achievement or psychosocial adjustment (these outcomes were apparently not measured), the PSM did seem to relieve the system of unnecessary and burdensome bureaucracy and allowed it to redeploy resources in a more child-centered than regulation-centered manner. What is appealing, moreover, is that this more individualized approach does not assume that just because an intervention shows promise in a randomized trial, it will work equally well for all students. The system is sufficiently flexible (theoretically) to appreciate and accommodate the considerable individual differences in student needs. Furthermore, the system regards teaching staff not as vessels to be trained to deliver a specified intervention with fidelity, but as active problem solvers who will engage on a collaborative basis to assess and address the problem of underperforming students. The PSM, however, requires extensive organizational management, staff education, and buy-in, since it is not just a technique but a change in school culture. Equally important, and relevant to the purpose of this book, it will require a theoretical approach that can provide an informed basis for understanding children and devising problem-solving strategies.

SPECIFIC LEARNING DISABILITY: R.I.P.?

Fifty years ago, the specific learning disability construct proved very successful as a basis for advocacy and a means to make real gains for children who struggled in school, but it is increasingly clear that the construct has mostly outlived its usefulness and is in decline in the United States. Practitioners increasingly behave *despite* the categorical diagnosis in order to provide children with what they need, rather than using the categorical diagnosis as a constructive means to advance the well-being of children. The emergence of new models with which experts are struggling, as evidenced by the 2005 IDEA, acknowledges this reality. Equally clear, the turmoil will continue for some time to come as new frameworks struggle into being within social contexts that will themselves inevitably continue to evolve.

As is further elaborated, however, since extant conceptual models of learning disabilities are essentially modular, they are likely inadequate to the task of understanding a *developmental* problem. Although these modular approaches certainly will continue to play an essential role, they will not, by themselves, rescue us from the definitional morass. Unfortunately, such approaches, if not complemented by a developmental perspective, will inevitably lead back to the same dilemmas that have plagued the field for so many years. *Parenthetically, although I will continue to use the term "learning disabilities" in this book, I do so for ease of understanding, with explicit recognition that part of the dilemma is inherent in the term itself and that it thus may be a placeholder for a new construct and terminology to be adopted in the future.*

The developmental paradigm elaborated in this book can provide the complementary theoretical perspective required to accommodate the real situations that children, parents, and teachers confront in their daily lives. Although it will surely bring its own set of dilemmas, it adds a dimension that has received little attention for too many years. It can more accurately model the actual phenomena, and it will profitably *complement* (not replace) existing modular strategies. It may be particularly well suited, moreover, to problem-solving models for managing children with learning problems. The term "developmental," however, sounds suspiciously vague. In order to be useful, it requires far more elaboration, especially as it relates to the learning disabilities dilemma.

Chapter 2

A Learning Disability Is a Developmental Problem

> Intelligence is an adaptation.
> —PIAGET (1963)

THE DEVELOPMENTAL PERSPECTIVE

The writings of the Swiss developmental psychologist and philosopher Jean Piaget triggered a transformation of the field of *child* psychology into *developmental* psychology. Through meticulous observation, Piaget discovered that the infant uses its experience to *construct* an understanding of the world. This view stood in stark contrast to prevalent beliefs that faculties of perception and cognition either matured on a preordained timetable or were registered by the environment on a blank slate, shaped by a complex system of stimulus and reward.

According to Piaget, from his or her earliest sensorimotor interactions with the immediate physical and social environment, the child *constructs* an understanding that transforms physical action and sensation into symbolic understanding. This understanding vastly extends the child's knowledge of, and capacity to interact with, the physical and social worlds. Intelligence is thus constructed through the repeated but expectable interactions of the child with the environment. Such learning is constrained by properties of the biological systems and of the environment (Piaget, 1963).

Accordingly, cognitive development, or intelligence, is essentially a process of *adaptation*, which Piaget understood to be the establishment of equilibrium between processes of assimilation and accommodation. Processes of *assimilation* incorporate data acquired from experience, and processes of *accommodation* modify internal cognitive schemata in relation to experiential transactions. These cognitive schemata are internally reorganized as the infant or child encounters new data that thrust the system into a state of disequilibrium. The continual process of moving toward a newly equilibrated state propels development and the associated construction of knowledge. Importantly, Piaget maintained that the "very concept of the object is far from being innate and necessitates a construction which is simultaneously assimilatory and accommodating" (1963, p. 7).

In the Piagetian view, the organism and the environment form an indissoluble entity. Elaborating on this position, Piaget made the following remarkable observation: "This is to admit the possibility of hereditary adaptations simultaneously *presupposing an action of the environment and a reaction of the organism other than the simple fixation of habits*" (1963, p. 18, emphasis added). In other words, biological systems have evolved to anticipate certain experiential regularities (e.g., objects fall down, caretakers speak). As we shall see in Chapter 3, the constancy of these expectable experiences can lead to an illusion of innateness. This intimate and ultimately indissoluble state of relationship between the organism and its environment is key to any developmental perspective. Importantly, it draws on both the Anglo-American empiricist and the European structuralist traditions to create an integrated framework that is informed by modern concepts in evolutionary and developmental biology.

Developmental neuroscience and genomics are beginning to provide empirical evidence for mechanisms that Piaget could only infer. Importantly, contemporary biological sciences also provide insight into specific constraints that can shape the adaptive processes that Piaget proposed. Piagetian theory, however, establishes basic principles that can inform a developmental paradigm for understanding and managing typical and atypical development, including learning problems. These can be summarized as follows:

1. The organism and the environment are intimately and inextricably engaged in a mutual transactional process such that *neither can exist independent of the other.*
2. These transactional processes are dynamic, resulting in the construction of cognitive structures that are continually transformed in an ongoing, nonlinear developmental process of adaptation to environmental demands.
3. Biologically based variations (e.g., genetic, neurological, endocrinological, experiential) are incorporated into this constructional process and integrated into the developing system, potentially affecting the system as a whole, not just a discrete component of cognitive functioning.

These core developmental principles have direct relevance to the learning disabilities dilemma. They can inform research, theory, and intervention, guiding a process of problem solving. Equally important, they can promote a more accurate understanding of individual children and their life narratives. Such a developmental approach entails consideration of simultaneously interacting spheres of functioning—brain, child, family, and society.

THE DEVELOPING BRAIN

Even though the human brain has a typical structural and functional architecture, each brain is a unique product of its genetic endowment and its specific experience. Because of the powerful influence of experience on brain development and the potentially infinite combinations of genes and gene expression, it follows that every brain will be unique, even within a spectrum of "normal," much like faces or fingerprints. No two individuals, even genetically identical twins have identical brains, even though they may exhibit strong similarities.

These individual brain differences may not be evident at the gross level—most people walk, talk, and think in distinctly human ways. At a subtler level, however, there is a vast array of dynamically interacting variations. These relatively subtle variations can gain greater significance as children encounter developmental challenges, even within the range of "normal."

To make a simple analogy, consider a basketball team. The rules of basketball pertain to every basketball game; the court has the same structure and dimensions; every team has members that fulfill each of the five key roles. This is the basic and expectable environmental constant that shapes the character of the team along with other contextual forces. Yet each game the team plays is unique. The game depends on the skill of the various players, how well they communicate with and anticipate one another, the particular court, the spirit of the fans, the physical and mental well-being of key players, the nature of the opposing team, and so on and so on. Moreover, experiences from one game can carry on to the next, transforming the team each time, so that by the end of the season, the team often looks very different than it did at the beginning. The transformations, however, are predictable to some extent, given the starting conditions. If the offensive players are relatively weak, the defensive players will try to compensate to prevent the opposition from gaining access to the basket. Drilling and coaching players to perfect their shooting and to execute plays are certainly necessary for a successful team. How the team fares, however, will ultimately be determined by the systemic inter-action of all the above factors, *including but not limited to specific skills.* Shooting practice is an essential tool, but it is only a tool.

In the same way, working with children to perfect their decoding skills, their fluency, and so forth, is undoubtedly necessary for them to become successful readers. But for many children with learning prob-lems, focused training on specific skills will not be sufficient to guar-antee a positive developmental outcome. Like a basketball coach, the educator or psychologist needs to appreciate the child at the system level in order to promote successful development. A developmental approach can be distinguished from a skill-based approach in this way, but nei-ther, by itself, is adequate to promote adaptive success.

In the range of human variety and adaptation, learning problems fall in the "subtle" category of variants (sometimes called high frequency–low impact). Moreover, functions do not develop separately but are mutually shaped by their interactions within an integrated system in a particu-lar environmental context. Children do not take out their reading brain when they go to school, their motor brain when they show up for soccer, and their social brain when they arrive at a birthday party. It is the same brain, functioning as a dynamic, developing *system* that encounters its world; it is continually influenced by these encounters and, in turn, influ-ences its world. Indeed, it is a tenet of Piagetian theory that cognitive schemata and their developmental transformations are manifest rela-tively consistently across functional domains.

This developmental perspective also asserts that the developing brain is very different from the adult brain in that its functions are not clearly organized in a "modular" fashion—that is, as discrete, encap-sulated functions. As the legendary Russian neuropsychologist A. R. Luria (1973) theorized in his *hierarchical model of function,* early and sometimes relatively subtle differences become elaborated in the course of development and incorporated systemically. Thus, in a child's brain a relatively small variation present early in development can, like a kernel or a seed, become manifest more globally. In an adult brain the elabo-rated skills have already been established, and functional organization is more modular. A similar injury in an adult brain will have more specific functional effects. Equally relevant, a developing brain may compen-sate for early maladaptive variations, sometimes constructing alternative pathways for accomplishing the same functional goal. Such compensa-tion, however, can incur a cost to the system as a whole. This distinction between *modular* and *developmental* approaches to functional brain development, further elaborated later, is essential to understanding the contribution of a developmental perspective.

THE DEVELOPING CHILD

The inherent tension between biologically based variation and social expectation emerges from the infant's first moments. Parents approach their newborn with expectations about feeding, sleeping, crying, fussing, and cuddling. Children typically exhibit regular developmental progressions in terms of motor and language development, state regulation, and so forth. However, a child may or may not conform to the baby manuals. Each child brings his or her unique temperament, regulatory capability, sensitivities, and ultimately personality into the world. Beyond the broad developmental trajectories, there is a vast array of individual differences, to which parents are acutely attuned. Not only does the child adapt to the structure and expectation of the parent, but equally important, the child shapes the parent's behavior. The parent–child dyad can be exquisitely sensitive to nuances in the behavior of each partner, as illustrated by the impact of maternal depression on the mother–infant interaction (Tronick & Reck, 2009). It is the dyad that develops as much as the child. Infants who are similarly irritable, may elicit different responses from different mothers, thus shaping, on a more individual basis, the longer-term consequences of that irritability. The way in which these subtle predispositions interact with the environment can influence the organization of the child's behavior in a variety of ways.

Children thus enter school with a wide variety of skills, personality characteristics, cognitive styles, experiences, and quirks. Nevertheless, there are shared cultural norms and expectations for their academic, cognitive, and social functioning, based on statistically informed models of "normal" or "typical" development. In elementary education in particular, the cultural norm is that all children should be able to meet a preconceived set of curricular standards for the age group, and that these skills should advance in lockstep. Thus, the third grader is expected to achieve certain curriculum-referenced standards in terms of reading comprehension, writing, and mathematical knowledge and computation. Although the majority of children will be able to conform to these expectations on most dimensions, a significant minority will not be able to do so, for a variety of reasons. Moreover, a child's neurocognitive profile will be carried across multiple situations, and experiences in one domain will have an impact on others. A child who has difficulty understanding complex language can struggle in mathematics, not because he or she cannot understand the concepts, but because he or she cannot understand the teacher!

The complexity of this problem is further compounded by the fact that children are constantly developing. As these powerful developmental processes unfold, children's capacities can change dramatically.

Despite superficial appearances, these changes typically do not proceed along a linear trajectory, as our second Piagetian principle emphasizes. Development is characterized by spurts and plateaus, involving a *systemic* reorganization of functions as new capacities are achieved. Understanding the causes of change is among the greatest challenges of developmental psychology (Johnson & Munakata, 2005). With development, functional systems become both better articulated and better integrated; changes in one functional system may spur reorganization of others. Therefore, the notion that there can be a "specific" developmental disorder of a skill such as reading or arithmetic lacks plausibility.

These developmental processes will have direct consequences for a child's cognitive and behavioral profile. Because of the processes of reorganization in the course of development, change can result in increased compensation in some circumstances or greater vulnerability in others. Some children may present with difficulties early in their school careers, whereas others begin to encounter difficulties later. Or a child may struggle in one aspect of the curriculum at one age and in other aspects later. Cognitive profiles that may appear dramatic at a young age may also become far less prominent with development, as compensatory systems become available, especially with effective intervention to modify the trajectory. Equally significant, well-constructed and empirically validated interventions may remediate a specific skill in the early years, only to have problems emerge in a related or other domain later. Given this complexity, it is hardly surprising that the challenge of deciding who does or does not "have" a disability has proven so daunting and often defeating.

THE ECOLOGICAL CONTEXT: A CHILD–WORLD SYSTEM

The Piagetian model seeks to explain universal regularities and consistencies in child development. Understanding the individual child, however, requires an appreciation of the child's adaptation within his or her particular social and cultural niche. The developmental psychologist Urie Bronfenbrenner was especially interested in these transactions between the child and both the proximal and distal environments. His model put the child at the center and posited various levels of interaction with the social system, ranging from the nuclear family to local institutions (schools and day care centers), to the community (neighborhood, town), and to the broader social, cultural, and economic environment (Bronfenbrenner, Morris, Damon, & Lerner, 1998). This ecological perspective is essential to understanding the meaning of learning problems. Although learning disorders clearly involve features of brain development that are associated with cognitive difficulties, the context within which the child's cognition is constructed is equally important. This context can include the language and cultural milieu provided by the immediate and extended family, family stressors, a parent's understanding of the child and interpretation of his or her actions, and, equally important, the impact of the child's responses on parent understandings and behavior. At the next level are factors such as the school environment, characteristics of particular teachers and peers, community resources, and attitudes toward differences. Of course, the legal system also impinges on the child with learning problems, as decisions are made about eligibility for potential support services. Local and state education budgets, for example, can be highly relevant to an individual child's development. Stricter or more liberal standards for eligibility for service provision, which can have repercussions in terms of the child's immediate academic environment, may shape teachers' perceptions of the child and the child's feelings toward the school and also have an impact on family functioning. School climate as well can be relevant; some school cultures are better equipped to manage differences than others or to provide a more structured and predictable environment. Likewise, teachers may themselves experience varying levels of support and appreciation or frustration and demoralization.

In addition, curricular expectations have changed substantially over the decades, such that today's children encounter academic challenges that were unimaginable for children being educated even several decades ago. Although it is, of course, important to maintain high standards and expectations for all students, it is equally important to recognize the potential consequences of such expectations and be prepared to deal with those consequences constructively. As expectations and demands change and escalate, and standards are adopted, so does the likelihood that more and more children will encounter "unexplained" learning problems.

As children emerge as outliers, especially with respect to their ability to meet criteria for academic performance, the question of a learning disability is often raised, setting into motion a series of clinical and legal involvements. Unlike other developmental disability diagnoses, however, learning disability exists as much in response to social demands as to any "defect" within the individual. To be perhaps overly simplistic, were it not for the cultural invention of text, there would be no diagnosis such as dyslexia. The same cannot be said of hearing or visual impairment.

Larger cultural values come into play as well. The U.S. education system is not unique in defining normality so as to marginalize individuals with less typical complements of cognitive strengths and weaknesses. Many other countries, however, have responded to the same dilemma simply by creating rigid classification systems that destine children to particular strata of society from a relatively young age, with potentially significant economic consequences. The American response, however, is shaped by a deep-seated value for the individual and for the individual's access to opportunity. In order to honor that value, its strategy for managing this phenomenon has been to develop a complex system of medical diagnoses and legal entitlements, and then to grapple with the increasingly unwieldy and often contentious system thus created. One symptom of this problem is the periodic introduction of a "new definition" that is intended to be superior to the one it replaced by identifying the children who *truly* have a learning disability. Although the American approach respects the individual and the individual's right to equal opportunity, it has created its own problems, spawning confusion, competition for limited educational resources to which a great many children might legitimately be entitled, inequities for children whose families do not have the knowledge or financial resources to pursue their potential entitlements, and parental expectations that sometimes cannot be met. Importantly, it has all too frequently led to acrimony between families and schools. All of these contextual factors will inevitably affect individual children because of the systemic nature of the phenomena.

The developmental emphasis on the intimate transactional process between an organism and its environment is compatible with the vast heterogeneity of profiles observed among children for whom a diagnosis of learning disability is entertained. This infinite potential for heterogeneity, as suggested earlier, explains to some extent why the diagnostic problem has proved so resistant to solution. For pragmatic political and legal reasons, the consensual definition must fit the broader disability model, paralleling the physical disabilities. Within this framework, it makes sense to conceptualize the diagnosis as a defect in a specific component of cognition, just as visual or hearing impairment implicates a specific component of sensation. Unfortunately, however, the clinical picture is often difficult to reconcile with this conceptualization, precisely because there is so much heterogeneity and because there can be so many routes to a final common pathway of "troubles." Equally important, the extent and manifestation of the problem, as Bronfenbrenner suggested, will inevitably be a function of the context, or "world," within which the child finds him- or herself, the child–world system (Bernstein & Waber, 1990). The family, the classroom, the curriculum, the school, the community, the legal and economic constraints, and social expectations—all of these constitute the world to which the child must adapt and, equally important, that must reciprocally adapt to the child.

The power of the interaction between the child and the world can be difficult to perceive in the contemporary moment, in which we make fixed assumptions about the world that we inhabit and see learning problems as residing within the child. However, the child–world interaction becomes much easier to perceive within a historical perspective. The social and economic meaning of childhood in the United States has evolved dramatically over just the past century, and of course it continues to evolve today. In the 19th century, a child's labor was essential to the economic survival of his or her family; in today's world, parents understand that if a child does not possess facility with symbolic material (i.e., text and computation), that child's ability to enter the workforce and support his or her own family economically will be compromised. Child labor is strictly regulated, and society places high value on attending school and achieving educational success. School success, in short, holds far more significance for contemporary children than it did in the past. This natural social evolution is obviously not frozen in place, but will continue to evolve and affect how children with heterogeneous cognitive capacities and profiles interact with their worlds. The interaction itself is a continually evolving process, depending not only on the child, but on the expectations and goals of schooling.

The Child–World Interaction in Historical Context

In his chronicle of childhood in America, *Huck's Raft*, social historian Stephen Mintz (2004) provides perspective on contemporary understandings about the meaning of childhood and schooling. In 19th-century America, only a small minority of children enjoyed the middle-class ideal of a slow and nurtured development to which we aspire for most American children today. For the growing middle class, schooling extended dependency and allowed children to enter the employment pool later in life. At the same time, however, the Industrial Revolution forced poorer families to put their children to work, effectively expanding the practice of child labor.

It is no accident that what is generally regarded as the first medical report of dyslexia concerned a boy from an upper-class background. English physician Pringle-Morgan (1896) described the perplexing case of Percy, a 14-year-old boy, who had had the advantage of schooling and tutors since he was 7 years of age, but he could not read or write. Percy was competent in arithmetic and thought to be bright but could not learn to read. Pringle-Morgan reported that Percy could not learn to spell the name of his father's house, an indication of his social status. At the time, universal literacy was by no means expected, but within an upper-class social rank, literacy was the norm. Hence, the boy's striking inability to conform to that norm became a matter of great concern, eventually resulting in a new medical diagnosis, "developmental dyslexia." Since working-class English children had no need to read in order to fulfill their economic role as laborers, such a diagnosis would not have surfaced in that social stratum.

By the dawn of the 20th century, schooling and literacy were still far from universal, even in democratic America, despite the efforts of school reformers. School attendance was far more prevalent in the middle than in the working classes, especially at the high school level. Literacy was not a cultural expectation in the working classes, since their labor did not require it and parents did not model literacy for their children. As the 20th century progressed, child labor declined, especially in the North, where compulsory education laws were the norm and waves of immigration provided a growing supply of cheap adult labor so that child labor was no longer so essential to the economy. Still, immigrant children were less likely to attend high school than their native-born peers, and child labor continued to flourish in the South to satisfy the need for cheap labor in the textile mills. Yet even though grammar school attendance had increased significantly by the early 20th century, only a fifth of students of high school age actually attended school. Moreover, *only 10% actually graduated high school*, an astonishingly low number by contemporary standards (Caplow, Bahr, Modell, & Chadwick, 1996; Mintz, 2004). Rather than attending school, most American teenagers came from working-class backgrounds and were employed as wage earners.

Significantly, for purposes of our discussion, political advocacy for universal education, laws against child labor, and school attendance brought many more students from diverse backgrounds into the schools for longer periods of time (Doris, 1987). Not only were children from the laboring classes now required to attend school, but there were large numbers of immigrant children who were not native English speakers, especially in the cities. This larger and more diverse student population soon resulted in large groups of schoolchildren who were falling behind their peers. By 1911, more than a third of children in the public schools was classified as "laggards" (Doris, 1987). From this social mix emerged a need for what came to be known as "special education." Until that time, children, especially those from the working classes, who did not easily acquire literacy, simply stopped going to school and entered the workforce, so there was no need to devote resources to educating them.

In the progressive era, however, mission-oriented educators were eager to serve and to educate the children of the working classes. Moreover, talented women who were unable to enter other professions often became teachers, and many applied their energies eagerly to this project. From this situation emerged educational structures that are easily recognized in contemporary schools—the graded organization of the general education curriculum and segregated classes for those who lag behind.

The former included tracking, in which children's abilities were assigned to slower or faster tracks based on perceived ability, but often with considerable flexibility (Doris, 1987).

School attendance was further boosted by the Great Depression of the 1930s. The economic collapse served to remove working-class children from the labor force in order to free up jobs for adults. In the midst of the Depression, more than half of all 17-year-olds were attending school, a dramatic shift from enrollment patterns earlier in the century. This higher rate of school attendance among adolescents, in turn, changed attitudes toward high-school-age children, leading to a longer period of economic and psychological dependence and expectations for greater academic achievement (Mintz, 2004).

The curriculum and culture of schools had also evolved. Under the influence of progressive educators such as John Dewey, leaders in public education sought to make schooling relevant for their students. They rejected the private school model where the primary goal of high school was to educate students for a liberal arts college education. Rather, they opted for more practical curricula, stressing vocational skills, civics, and health education along with basic reading, writing, and mathematics skills.

Eventually, however, there was a backlash to progressive influences in education—American schools were seen as falling short and American children as inadequately taught. In 1955 Rudolph Flesch published his classic book, *Why Johnny Can't Read,* in which he advocated phonics and scorned the "look–say" method. The cover assured readers: "Use this book and you can teach your child to read in six weeks." The book's title became a rallying cry for a new generation of education reformers. Then, in October 1957, the U.S.S.R. launched *Sputnik* and a month later sent a dog into space. The educational system, especially progressive education, was viewed as a major reason the U.S. lagged behind the Russians in technological advancement. The more practically oriented brand of education offered by high schools in the 1930s and 1940s was blamed for the failure. There was a call to increase academic rigor, not only in reading but also in science and math. Education became a primary focus of the nation's Cold War anxiety, and the more progressive, child-centered educational philosophy took a back seat (Mintz, 2004).

When Samuel Kirk coined the term "learning disability" in 1963, just a few years after the launch of *Sputnik*, there was growing pressure to raise standards in U.S. schools. There was also a social consensus that children belonged in school and not in the workforce. In the early 1960s, upwards of 60% of American children were graduating from high school. Moreover, it was becoming apparent, especially to the middle classes, that school success would be essential to future economic success.

Over the past century, powerful economic forces have changed the complexion of labor in the United States and other developed countries. These economic forces have shaped educational expectations and conditions. Figure 2.1 shows changes in the distribution of categories of work over the past century and a half. In the late 19th century, the lion's share of employment was in agriculture, fisheries, and mining—jobs that required physical labor but little in the way of symbolic skills. In the 20th century, that sector was supplanted by manufacturing—jobs that were often less physically demanding and required basic literacy and numeracy, but were nonetheless essentially manual labor. In the latter half of the century, however, the proportion of jobs in that sector declined, replaced by information-intensive and technical jobs, with much of the rest of the economy populated by less well paying service-sector jobs. The shift from agriculture and then manufacturing to information management and technology has had direct consequences for schools. In the late 19th and early 20th centuries, a head of household, aided by adolescent children, could support a family without a high school education. In the mid-20th century, reflecting the gains of organized labor, many manufacturing jobs paid well enough to support a middle-class lifestyle. In the early 21st century, however, that is no longer the case. Families and schools feel intense pressure to educate children for a labor force that can sustain the economy and provide the means to support a middle-class family. A young person who does not complete high school and even college can be at a significant lifelong disadvantage.

The long espoused goal of universal literacy, however, still remains more a goal than an achievement. In a study carried out by the Organization for Economic Cooperation and Development (OECD), the International Adult Literacy Survey was administered to representative samples of adults in the OECD countries (OECD, 2000), the most developed in the world. Fewer than 60% of American adults met minimum standards of literacy—that is, had skills sufficient to cope with the demands of everyday life and work in a complex, information-based society. Thus, 40% of adults did not possess adequate literacy to succeed in the society in which they lived. The statistics are only slightly better among adolescents, indicating that this problem is not simply a generational one.

As the goal posts are advanced, in keeping with social and economic demands, it is likely that more individuals will be identified as deficient. Equally important, as good-paying jobs that require physical or manual labor become scarcer, the pressure from families and social institutions to assure advanced literacy and numeracy will continue to grow, and the intensity of interest in education and school achieve-

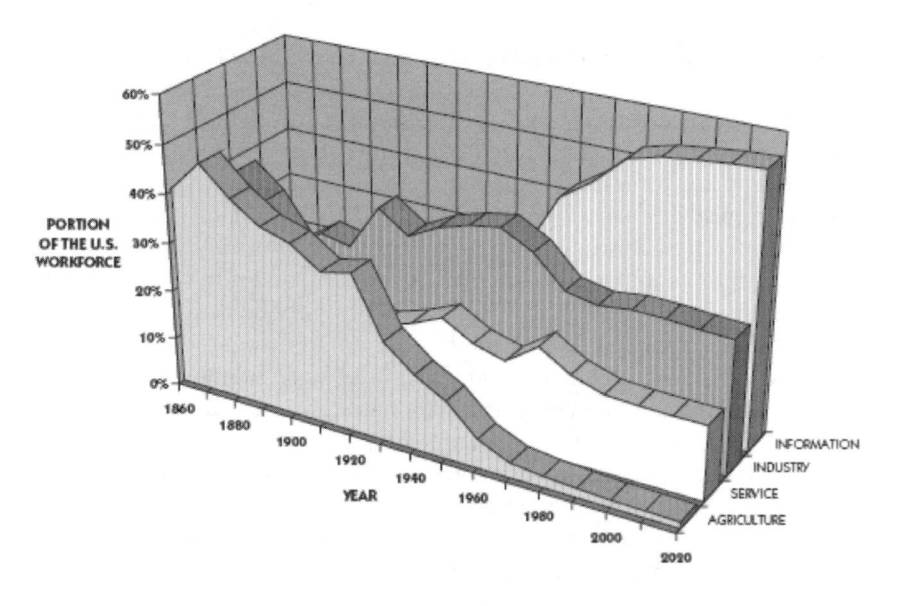

FIGURE 2.1. Proportion of the U.S. workforce engaged in agriculture, service, industry, and information from 1860 and projected to 2020. From Nilles, J. M. (1999, August 30). *Electronic commerce and new ways of working: Penetration, practice and future development in the U.S.A. and around the world.* Copyright by JALA International. Reprinted by permission.

ment will escalate. The OECD statistics suggest that nearly 40% of our schoolchildren are potential candidates for a diagnosis of learning disability. Considerable additional resources would be required were all those children to be served appropriately under existing disability and special education models. It is hardly surprising, therefore, that identification criteria continue to be so hotly debated. Moreover, despite rapid gains in the first half of the 20th century, high school graduation rates peaked at about 70% in the late 1960s and have not improved significantly since then (Seastrom, Hoffman, Chapman, & Stillwell, 2005), indicating potential risk for a learning disability diagnosis for a large segment of the population.

THE SOCIAL CONTEXT OF LEARNING DISABILITY DETERMINATION

From its early days, the critique has been leveled that the learning disability diagnosis is one of the middle and upper classes. There is no doubt that this was true, especially in the early years. Advocacy groups are primarily powered by more affluent families who have knowledge and resources and who are culturally adept at advocating for their children's needs. Sociologist Annette Lareau (2003), in her book *Unequal Childhoods*, characterizes the childrearing style of higher-socioeconomic-status American parents as *concerted cultivation*, which she contrasts with that of lower-income parents, which she calls *natural development*. Inherent in these contrasting styles are parents' attitudes toward schools as institutions. With their more activist stance, higher-socioeconomic-status families feel comfortable challenging schools and their bureaucracies to respond if they feel their child is not being properly educated. Lower-socioeconomic-status families, especially new immigrants, can be more deferential, assuming that teachers and other school personnel are professionals who know best about educating their children. The fierce parental advocacy that procures special education support for more economically advantaged youngsters, therefore, may not be exercised as energetically on behalf of children from lower socioeconomic environments or for children whose parents may not have the cultural skills or economic means to advocate. Critics have also argued that in lower-income communities special education can become a repository for children with behavior problems, more typically from minority groups, often because few other options are available (Oswald, Coutinho, & Best, 2002). Indeed, the social context within which a child is schooled is potentially a significant determinant of learning disability identification, again illustrating the salience of the "world" component of the system. In more advantaged school districts, where the general level of achievement is high, a child who performs in the average range may garner more support and even special education resources than a child whose overall level of performance is lower but who is from a less advantaged district where the global need is greater.

Significantly, the legal definition of *learning disability* includes the requirement that the problem is not primarily the result of "environmental disadvantage." Thus, a child from a suburban middle-class environment whose reading is a year below grade level may be entitled to special education services, whereas a child from a lower-income environment with the same cognitive profile may be entitled only to Title I services, typically delivered by teachers without special education training, even though the two children's problems may be phenomenologically comparable. Although such a distinction may have made sense 30 years ago, we now know that brain development is materially affected by experience. By the age of 3, for example, children of low-income mothers on welfare have heard only one-fourth as many spoken words as those of high-income professional mothers (Hart & Risley, 1995). Developmentally, the experiential differences are reflected not only in early language but eventually in reading skill (Hart & Risley, 2003).

The potential adverse impact of class on child development is not confined to lower-income children, however. The psychologist Suniya Luthar has written extensively on the mental health of children from more affluent backgrounds (e.g., Luthar & Latendresse, 2005). Although she set out to study children from economically disadvantaged circumstances, she soon discovered that many children of affluence were, in fact, in greater emotional distress than their less economically advantaged peers. Academic pressure is a major source of stress and psychological morbidity among these youngsters. Thus contextually, even though a child in a higher-income setting may exhibit academic and/or cognitive problems that seem mild on an objective basis, the psychosocial consequences can be significant, and so these need to be regarded seriously as well in relation to longer-term adaptive success.

Learning Disability Internationally

From an international perspective, the concept of a learning disability is highly dependent on the social and economic context within which schooling occurs. In Africa, where there may be 40 students in a class, teacher training is not well developed, and "under-the-tree" classes are still held in many places, the concept of a learning disability and special education is nascent in the universities but very rarely recognized or implemented in practice (Abosi, 2007). The concept of a learning disability is emergent and recognized in India, where the goal of universal education is normative and economic development is a national goal, but only limited resources are available for such children, who are greatly underserved (Crawford, 2007; Karande et al., 2007). In China, where unskilled labor has driven economic growth and education is essentially an elitist enterprise, the concept of a learning disability, or even autism, is not yet recognized; special education services are mandated only for children with deafness, blindness, or significant mental retardation (McLoughlin, Zhou, & Clark, 2005). In other Asian countries such as South Korea and Japan, however, that have a substantial middle class, thriving democracies and highly developed economies, the concept is better recognized but still emerging and gaining social acceptance on a cultural basis (Jung, 2007). Similarly, in Taiwan, there is a special education law modeled after that in the United States, but few school staff to implement it, and fewer than 1% of students are even identified (Tzeng, 2007). In the United Kingdom, the term "dyslexia" is widely used to refer to a severe reading problem, but other cognitive issues that could interfere with school adaptation are less frequently accorded official recognition. The term "learning disabled" is reserved for children whom Americans would consider to have borderline intellectual functioning.

Nowhere in the world is the learning disability construct as well developed and complex as in the United States. As we in the United States continue to stress universal standards of achievement and opportunity for all children, and as parents experience growing anxiety about the economic prospects of the next generation and seek to exercise legal rights, we should anticipate a continuing increase in the numbers of children for whom concerns about learning problems, most of which are legitimate, will be raised. At the same time, available resources for special education may be shrinking in response to economic pressures. In light of these particularly American social contextual pressures, it is inevitable that the stresses associated with the learning disability dilemma will only intensify, demanding better solutions than those that are currently available.

BARTHOLOMEW AND ELIZABETH: A TALE OF TWO WORLDS

To illustrate the power of the context in making sense of learning problems, consider the following scenario. Bartholomew Simpson sits in a fifth-grade classroom in a suburban Midwestern community where he lives with his parents and little sister, Elizabeth. His father, Herman, has a successful business selling flooring materials; his mother, Meg, was trained as a teacher but now works part-time as an administrator in the family business. Bartholomew struggles to make sense of the words on a page. With the benefit of early reading intervention, he can read the words, but it is hard work for him, and he does not particularly enjoy it. He gets passing grades, but even when he invests effort, his grades tend toward the bottom of his class. He has come to accept that he is not so bright and is less and less inclined to work hard at school since the prospects for success are slim anyway. When he needs to compose a short book report on a science text, he has trouble figuring out what to write and how to get the right words on the page. At home, he loves to play video games and to explore the outdoors. In school, however, he is increasingly misbehaving, not doing his work, and distracting other children.

The teacher suggests to the Simpsons that there may be "something more going on" with Bartholomew, and urges them to consult the pediatrician about whether he might have ADHD. Thus begins the familiar series of evaluations, and Bartholomew questions himself further. "What is wrong with me? Is something wrong with my brain? Why am

I dumb?" Eventually, it is declared that Bartholomew has ADHD, inattentive subtype, and dyslexia. A trial of stimulant medication is recommended and Bartholomew is once again enrolled in special education. He leaves the classroom every morning for 45 minutes in a reading support group, but continues to struggle with the rest of his subjects. Although he is still not so happy about going to school, he feels somewhat better about reading and is not quite so lost and helpless.

Bartholomew's little sister Elizabeth, in contrast, has already earned accolades as a star student by the second grade, infuriating and humiliating Bartholomew and creating ongoing tension within the family. She and Bartholomew will never be close. She breezes through school, apparently with relatively little effort.

Bartholomew goes on to middle school with his individualized education plan. He is mainstreamed for most of his subjects but continues to see the reading specialist three times a week. School remains basically boring and unappealing, and he becomes sullen and increasingly withdrawn. At home, he disappears into his room for hours to play video games or surf the Internet. In high school he eventually is tracked in the lower academic groups, where he finds the curriculum manageable but uninspiring. He continues to have periodic behavior problems, occasionally experimenting with drugs and alcohol, but never to such an extent that he is unable to attend school or to function in his typical, somewhat disengaged, fashion. Finally, to everyone's relief, Bartholomew graduates high school and, like most of his classmates, he heads to college.

His sister Elizabeth's stellar record earns her admission to a competitive private liberal arts college in the East, where she flourishes. After graduating, she spends 2 years working for a nonprofit agency that provides legal aid to new immigrants, and she then goes on to law school, where she meets her future husband. She becomes a successful lawyer, ultimately nominated to be a judge, and goes on to have a very satisfying career with many accomplishments.

Bartholomew spends several years in the state college system, where he is moderately successful but still not particularly interested or satisfied. Finally, he decides to take a break after so many years of school struggles. With his parents' blessing, he takes a leave and seeks full-time employment. Through a friend of the family, he finds a job with a company that installs heating, ventilation, and air conditioning (HVAC) systems. There he discovers that he is not as dumb as he thought—in fact, he actually has a knack for the more technically complicated installations, quickly earning the respect of his boss and coworkers. Bartholomew never returns to the state college; he enrolls instead in a program at a nearby community college to earn a certificate as an installer. Suddenly, he discovers that he is eager to go to class, and for the first time, he is energetic and engaged in school. Although he has to invest effort at times to read the technical manuals, he does not mind.

Within 5 years he has moved to a supervisory role, teaching younger workers the trade. He marries and settles down happily to raise his family in a town not far from where he grew up. Despite his successes in the world of work, however, he continues to think of himself as unintelligent because he was not "good" at school. Nevertheless, his life is now satisfying, he is supporting his family well, and he takes pleasure from his accomplishments and the respect with which he is now regarded.

Suppose we project these children back to an earlier time in our country's history to see how they develop within their "world." Let's assume that Bartholomew was born in the late 1860s to a couple who farmed and raised livestock in the Midwest. He was the third of six children but only one of three who survived infancy. From the time they were 7 or 8 years old, Bartholomew and his brother and sister, like most local children, spent much of their time performing chores on the farm and in the home. Bartholomew helped to care for the livestock, to carry water from the well, to plant and harvest crops, and to tend the family's small apple orchard. Indeed, without their labor, the farm would not have been viable.

A one-room school had been established in town, and Bartholomew was enrolled, attending more regularly in the winter months when there was less need for his labor on the farm. The Simpson children walked several miles into town each day to attend school, but when the weather was harsh they stayed home. Bartholomew, like many of the other boys, bridled at the tedium and drill of schoolwork. He spent much of his time in school pursuing mischief with his friends and waiting for the snow to melt so that he could spend more time on the farm and exploring the outdoors. By the time he was 10, he could sound out some words, write his name and simple sentences, and do basic calculations, enough to get by. His younger sister Elizabeth, however, loved school. She grasped reading easily and by the time she was 8 or 9 years of age, she was devouring whatever books her teacher could find for her.

Out of school, Bartholomew disappeared into the barn, tinkering with the tools and fussing over the animals. He had a knack for farm equipment and fixing things, and he loved caring for the animals. When Bartholomew was 12, his father arranged an apprenticeship for him with a blacksmith in town, and he was no longer expected to attend school. Because it took so long for him to walk back and forth from town to the farm, he went to live with the blacksmith and his wife, but frequently visited the farm and pitched in wherever he was needed, spending more time there in planting and harvest seasons. Bartholomew's father could not afford for both boys to leave home and apprentice, but the farm would not support everyone as the children grew up. The money Bartholomew could eventually earn as a smith would help the family make ends meet.

Bartholomew was a quick study, learning the trade easily and soon becoming a valued member of the blacksmith's household. The blacksmith increasingly relied on Bartholomew to operate his business. By the time he was 16, Bartholomew had taken over much of the work. Bartholomew's rudimentary reading and math skills were more than adequate to keep track of accounts and manage the business. Moreover, his work was valued and in demand in the area, so it was clear that he would earn a good livelihood in his trade. When the blacksmith could no longer work, Bartholomew took over the business and was very successful, becoming a well-respected citizen of his town and county.

Elizabeth, the scholar, spent whatever time she could helping the teacher in the schoolhouse until she herself married and had to devote herself full time to managing her own household on a nearby farm and raising her family. She loved her books with a passion, but her duties as a mother and wife left little time for reading. She also loved her children, but she grew disconsolate as she became increasingly isolated on the farm and worn down by the tedium of chores. She was often sick with headaches, spending days at a time in a darkened room, and even when she was pain free, she tired easily. The doctors tried various medicines and cures, but with little success. For the rest of her life, Elizabeth was periodically confined to bed. She came to be known as a sickly and disabled woman, and many remembered with sadness the lively young girl they had known.

Although the stories of Bartholomew and Elizabeth present an extreme case, spanning centuries, they illustrate the importance and fluidity of social context. Assumptions that are true today are different from assumptions that were true even a decade or two ago. More troubling, assumptions made in one town often differ substantially from those made in a town a few miles away. These assumptions can have direct impact on the lives of children. This contextual perspective helps to explain why the "specific learning disability" diagnosis has been so elusive.

DIAGNOSING THE DEFICIT
OR DIAGNOSING THE INTERACTION?

The developmental perspective views the organism and the environment as a seamless system. Thus, a learning problem is not a discrete entity that resides within the child, but a problem in the interaction between the child and the child's world. From this more systemic perspective, the learning disability diagnosis is best understood as *a social construction that serves to correct for the inherent incompatibility between* normally occurring *biological heterogeneity and socially determined expectations*. It is not a problem of *disability* but of *adaptation*. In this developmental paradigm, the location of the problem similarly does not lie in a defect or disability *in the child*, but in the *interaction between the child and the world*. That is, the problem is located in the dynamic relationship between a particular child's complement of skills and the particular environment in which that child is developing. It is precisely because the phenomena associated with learning disability reflect a *failed interaction* rather than a discrete defect in the child that implementation of the legal protections and entitlements has been so troubled and contentious.

This developmentally informed child–world notion (Bernstein & Waber, 1990) is not novel. Two decades ago, Gerald Senf (1987) suggested that the learning disability diagnosis is a "sponge" that serves to wipe up life's spills. Although the metaphor may have been inept, it was also prescient of the dilemma that was to ensue for the following decades, as researchers and policymakers struggled to find the perfect but elusive formula that would solve the dilemma of identification. Senf's view that a learning disability reflects a mismatch between the child's competencies and socially determined expectations, however, never received serious consideration. This lack of attention was largely attributable to the overriding pragmatic need to define a diagnosis in such a way that it retained its disability status, compatible with the requirements of the legal system. To admit that *learning disability* is essentially indefinable—the most expeditious conclusion from a neurodevelopmental and clinical standpoint—would risk losing the enormous gains achieved for children who once languished in an educational system that erroneously and cruelly branded them as cognitively limited or lazy. Yet by allowing legal requirements to dominate the direction of research, theory, and practice, we have ceded our ability as educators, scientists, and clinicians to honestly describe the phenomenology of "learning disability." The domination of legal requirements has also condemned the field to an endless preoccupation with the search for the perfect and inevitably elusive definition. After so many years of struggling to make sense of the phenomena, however, we may have reached a historical moment that allows us to reconsider learning problems with a more informed scientific understanding of relevant developmental processes. The next chapter reviews some of what science is telling us about developmental processes and the implications of that knowledge for understanding learning disabilities.

Chapter 3

A Developmental Science Perspective on Learning Disabilities

Development itself is the key to understanding
developmental disorders.
                    —KARMILOFF-SMITH (1998)

Although the specific learning disability diagnosis has rarely
been considered developmentally, it is not unique among developmental disorders in this respect. Many neuropsychological studies of developmental disorders, including learning disabilities, have adopted what
has been called a "static neuropsychological approach" (Oliver, Johnson, Karmiloff-Smith, & Pennington, 2000) that is essentially imported
from adult neuropsychology, which has historically adopted a modular
theoretical framework. In studies of adults, neuropsychologists correlate
an injury to a particular brain structure with compromise of a specific
cognitive or behavioral function. For example, a stroke in the language
areas of the left hemisphere correlates with aphasia, the loss of language
capacity. It has often been assumed, as a corollary, that cognitive competencies are correlated with the same brain structures in children as those
identified by the adult brain-damage studies. Accordingly, acquisition of
a specific skill is taken as evidence of maturation of the correlated brain
region.

In general, however, developmental time or processes tend not to
be especially relevant to these correlations. Equally important, a deficit is presumed to be discrete or circumscribed, leaving the remaining
"spared" functions relatively unscathed. Prevailing contemporary con-

ceptualizations of learning disability clearly reflect this orientation. Reading impairment, or dyslexia, is understood as a *specific* deficit in reading skill in the context of intact cognition. Moreover, this specificity is seen as relatively invariant developmentally. Although the challenge of the reading task may evolve over time, the problem is assumed to be *restricted to reading* throughout development. It follows from such a conceptual model that the appropriate response to dyslexia or reading impairment is to develop and implement evidence-based interventions to "fix" the deficit, thereby solving the problem. In reality, as has been discussed, the clinical experience of these children can be much more complex and varied, involving issues well beyond decoding single words or even comprehending sentences. Here is where a developmental perspective can be helpful.

In a developmental model, skills are not hardwired in the brain, like a light bulb that can be switched on or off. Rather, skills are constructed systemically *as a function of the ongoing interaction of genes, organism, and environment over developmental time.* Cognitive capacities become increasingly distinct from one another as a function of these developmental processes, eventually taking on the more modular organization seen in adults. Equally important, development is *systemic*; that is, various functions develop in interaction with one another and in interaction with the environment in ways that are ultimately inseparable. Thus, the developmental approach demands attention to the broader systemic context within which any particular skill evolves. As the science discussed in the next section shows, similar genetic information can have multiple phenotypic outcomes, depending on a multitude of experiential influences; by the same token, similar phenotypic outcomes can arise from multiple causal routes.

THE BIOLOGICAL BASES
OF LEARNING (READING) DISORDERS

Observers have long recognized that learning problems run in families (Stephenson, 1907). Rutter, Graham, and Yule (1970) observed that children with reading problems came from families that themselves had an elevated prevalence of reading problems. More recently, scientists are providing sophisticated genetic data to substantiate such clinical observations. Much of contemporary scientific research in this area has been motivated by the vision of a biological marker that could identify a specific learning disorder before the child has experienced failure; the child could then be treated with evidence-based interventions, which would ultimately normalized his or her brain function. To unpack the biological bases of learning disabilities, researchers have concentrated their efforts in two key areas: genetics and neuroscience.

In the process, however, they paradoxically encounter the same fundamental challenge that proved so vexing clinically and that the biological studies were intended to inform. Specifically, because of the very heterogeneous clinical presentations of children with learning problems, it is very difficult to decide who, in fact, "has" a learning disability. As a result, it is by no means obvious who should be eligible for studies and what aspects of their cognition should be studied.

To solve this dilemma, biological researchers have followed the lead of cognitive researchers, sidestepping the issue of defining a "learning-disabled" child. Instead, they have focused almost exclusively on specific discrete skills, generally reading and, to a much lesser extent, math (Shaywitz et al., 2004; Silani et al., 2005; Stanberry et al., 2006). The neuroscientific study of *learning disability*, therefore, for all intents and purposes, transformed itself into the neuroscientific study of *reading skill*. With this focus, several decades of work have produced considerable progress, to the point that reading skill can now actually be linked to genetic markers at the molecular level.

STATISTICAL STUDIES OF THE GENETICS OF READING DISORDERS

In 1983 Smith and colleagues (Smith, Kimberling, Pennington, & Lubs, 1983) published a paper that ignited interest in the genetic contribution to reading disorders. By applying statistical genetic techniques to the study of extended families, they linked the dyslexic profile to a site on chromosome 15. Since that time, a number of other studies have also pointed to genetic loci on chromosome 15, although results vary in their specifics (Grigorenko et al., 1997; Rabin et al., 1993; Schulte-Körne et al., 1998; Smith, Kimberling, & Pennington, 1991).

The most intuitively compelling evidence that reading skill has genetic roots, however, comes from twin studies. These studies compare *monozygotic* twins, who develop from one fertilized egg that has split, with *dizygotic* twins, who develop from two separate fertilized eggs. Monozygotic twins share 100% of their DNA; dizygotic twins share only 50% of their DNA, like other sibling pairs. If a trait such as dyslexia has a genetic basis, the concordance, or co-occurrence, of the trait will be significantly higher in monozygotic than in dizygotic twins. In 1987 researchers from the Colorado Twin Study reported that this is indeed the case: The concordance for dyslexia was 68% for monozygotic twins, but only 38% for dizygotic twins (DeFries, Fulker,

& LaBuda, 1987). It is worth noting, however, that among monozygotic twins who share *all* their DNA, co-occurrence of dyslexia fell well short of 100%. This indicates that other factors must be highly relevant as well. Monozygotic twins who are *discordant* for reading ability can thus be of great clinical and theoretical interest, since they can highlight potential environmental influences. Later in this book we shall meet just such a pair of twins.

The Colorado studies provided substantial impetus for more ambitious studies on the genetic bases of reading disorder. A method commonly used in more recent research is called "linkage analysis." Linkage studies use complex statistical methods to detect associations between specific genetic locations and particular traits. Using data from extended families or from twins, geneticists compare the likelihood that the observed pattern would have occurred if the trait and the genetic location on the chromosome were associated, versus the likelihood that they were not associated. The ratio between these two likelihood statistics is called an LOD (likelihood of difference) score. The higher the LOD score, the more likely it is that the genotype and the clinical phenotype are indeed associated. Another common technique, called "association analysis," searches for populationwide correlations between a trait, or phenotype, and specific genes. Collectively, these statistically based studies have implicated sites on chromosomes 2, 3, 6, 15, and 18, with 6 and 15 being the most consistent (Fisher & Francks, 2006).

Plomin and Kovas (2005), however, have cautioned that the genes associated with reading are more likely to be "generalists" than specific. That is, genes that affect one component of the disability, such as phonological awareness in reading, will also affect other components of reading and, moreover, are systematically associated with other cognitive skills, such as oral language and even mathematics. Precisely what these genes do, therefore, remains a problematic research concern, and the likelihood that there is a specific "reading gene" is thus questionable.

MOLECULAR GENETIC STUDIES OF READING DISORDERS

With the advent of molecular genetics, scientists are no longer limited to statistical models but can actually pinpoint genes and measure their biological activity. The mapping of the human genome and the availability of sophisticated molecular genetic techniques have allowed researchers to narrow their search from regions of chromosomes to specific candidate genes. Molecular genetic tools, therefore, can reveal reliable associations of specific genes with reading impairment. Even more important, they can provide a glimpse into the actual biological mechanisms by which gene function affects brain development, potentially resulting eventually in reading disorders.

Several laboratories working independently have linked dyslexia to a gene labeled *DCDC2*, which sits on chromosome 6 (Burbridge et al., 2008; Meng et al., 2005; Paracchini et al., 2006; Schumacher et al., 2006). Identification of this gene has led to studies exploring how *DCDC2* actually functions in the brain. Meng and colleagues (2005) examined human brain tissue samples to find out where the *DCDC2* gene was "expressed"—that is, in what regions of the brain it exerts a biological effect on neuronal function. The *DCDC2* gene, it turns out, is actually expressed in some of the same brain regions known to be associated with reading (i.e., the inferior and medial temporal cortex). Regions not associated with reading (e.g., amygdala, hypothalamus, hippocampus), however, also showed high levels of *DCDC2* expression. Another gene that has been repeatedly associated with reading ability in children and adults, *KIAA0319* (Harold et al., 2006; Paracchini et al., 2006, 2008), is likewise expressed in many regions throughout the adult human brain (Velayos-Baeza, Toma, Paracchini, & Monaco, 2008) and likely many regions in the developing brain. This more diffuse pattern of expression is, in fact, more typical of gene expression in the brain, where a single gene affects multiple structures (Oliver et al., 2000). Thus, it would be misleading to call *DCDC2* or *KIAA0319* "reading" genes, since they theoretically could be associated with many functions that may bear little direct or even indirect relation to reading. Moreover, as more and more researchers become involved in this area, inconsistencies have surfaced (de Kovel et al., 2008; Luciano et al., 2007). These inconsistencies are as likely to be related to the specific populations studied or to the criteria used to define dyslexia as to the genes themselves.

Since dyslexia is a developmental disorder, the role of these genes in early brain development is relevant. One of the basic mechanisms of structural brain development is *neuronal migration*. Neurons do not simply sprout in their appointed place; they are typically born on the surface of the ventricles (the fluid-filled cavities contained within the cerebral cortex) and then *migrate* outward to their target locations, guided largely by chemical stimuli. Like members of a college marching band at halftime, these newborn neurons can initially appear chaotic and undifferentiated, but as each seeks its target location, the more complex and organized mature brain structure takes shape. Neural migration is thus a crucial process for normal brain development, and disorders of migration can result in developmental disabilities, some quite severe.

When *DCDC2* expression was chemically blocked in the brains of prenatal rats, the effect was actually fairly subtle. Neurons in which

DCDC2 is typically expressed still moved toward their proper destination, but they did not migrate as far as they should. These subtle effects suggested that *DCDC2 modulates* neuronal migration but does not *control* it. This makes sense since the brains of individuals with dyslexia are grossly normal but may display subtle structural differences (Galaburda, 2002; Klingberg et al., 2000) consistent with the relatively mild functional effects seen in children with learning disabilities. Indeed, in mice, disruption of the gene that has been linked to reading is associated with abnormal migration, leading to areas of dystopia (i.e., clusters of neurons in the wrong location), similar to those Galaburda and associates demonstrated in the brains of dyslexic adults (Burbridge et al., 2008). These dystopic areas, however, were distributed throughout the cortex and, again, might be expected to affect multiple regions and thus functions. This accords with the developmental principle cited at the outset that functional variation in the developing organism is systemically expressed.

Gene expression, moreover, is not limited to early development: Genes are typically turned off and on throughout development, long after neuronal migration is complete. Moreover, as was discussed, a single gene can be expressed in many brain regions. What *DCDC2*, *KIAA0319*, and other genes linked to dyslexia actually do at later stages of development, during childhood and throughout adulthood, is not known. Even if the expression of this gene were to impair the potential for reading acquisition, it could well have other effects, beneficial or deleterious, that are not yet recognized. Moreover, within a developmental perspective, causal links are bidirectional. Harlaar, Dale, and Plomin (2007), for example, demonstrated that early reading skills are linked to reading exposure (i.e., children who read more easily read more), thereby leading to a developmental cascade of events that amplifies the genetic influence, recapitulating Stanovich's (1986) famous characterization of the "Matthew effect" in reading.

NEUROSCIENTIFIC STUDIES OF READING IMPAIRMENT

The search for sources of reading disability has been substantially advanced not only by molecular genetics but also by sophisticated techniques for creating visual images of brain structure. Structural imaging techniques such as segmentation and parcellation as well as diffusion tensor imaging allow scientists to quantify in great detail not only the size, shape, and volume of neuronal regions but the volume and organization of fibers connecting them. Functional magnetic resonance imaging (fMRI) provides information about which brain regions are active during mental task performance, and magnetoencephalography (MEG) and other electroencephalographic (EEG) techniques measure the precise timing of this activity. These technological achievements have revolutionized our understanding of how the brain processes information. Brain imaging techniques have been adopted enthusiastically by reading researchers to explore neural bases of typical and atypical reading acquisition and skill.

The prevailing theoretical rationale, which has guided many of these studies, is well summarized by Shaywitz and Shaywitz (2005). They write that the root cause of dyslexia is a deficit in the "phonologic module," which impairs the child's ability to segment words into their phonological components in order to link sounds to letters. Thus, the child has difficulty first in decoding the word and then in identifying it. They go on to explain that "the phonologic deficit is domain-specific; that is, it is *independent of other, non-phonologic abilities. In particular, the higher order cognitive and linguistic functions* ... such as general intelligence and reasoning, vocabulary and syntax are generally intact" (p. 1032, emphasis added). This "circumscribed" phonological deficit blocks access to higher-order processes and thereby blocks the ability to extract meaning from text. More recently, this theory has been updated as researchers have become more aware of the role of the left temporal–occipital region, where the visual and language areas are integrated. This area, at one time known as the "visual word form area," is thought to be fundamental for the development of reading fluency. According to the Shaywitz model, dysfunction in the phonological module has a downstream effect on the visual module. It is equally plausible, however, that the visual area is independently affected or that there is more widespread compromise of left-hemisphere regions related to language. Modifying their strictly modular view somewhat, Shaywitz and Shaywitz (2008) have more recently suggested that attentional processes play a functional role in reading as well, although their model still appears to view attention as a comorbid impaired module.

The initial wave of neuroimaging studies encountered considerable practical constraints. For example, techniques such as positron emission tomography (PET) involved exposures to radioactive substances and often required an ability to lie motionless in the bore of a scanner for long periods of time and to comply with task demands. Early studies were, therefore, carried out with adults with a history of poor reading, who were presumed to have developmental dyslexia. When neuroscientists began these studies, they had a fairly good idea about which brain regions were likely to distinguish dyslexic readers, based on decades of clinical observation of adults who had sustained brain injuries. Reading could be severely impaired by injuries to the left posterior region of the brain, involving the temporal, parietal, and occipital lobes (Pincus & Tucker, 1985).

In a pioneering study, Rumsey and her colleagues (1992) compared brain activation in men with and without dyslexia during a rhyming task, which required analysis of the component sounds of words (e.g., *cat* = /k/ + /at/). As expected, men with dyslexia exhibited less activation of the left temporal–parietal region. Since that time, numerous studies have implicated the same general regions in adults with developmental dyslexia, in terms of both brain structure (Eliez et al., 2000; Klingberg et al., 2000; Rumsey et al., 1997; Silani et al., 2005) and function (Horwitz, Rumsey, & Donohue, 1998; Paulesu et al., 1996, 2001; Shaywitz et al., 1998).

With the advent of fMRI, which does not entail ionizing radiation, it became possible to conduct neuroimaging studies with children. These studies similarly implicated the left posterior quadrant of the cerebral cortex in reading ability and disability (Georgiewa et al., 2002; Shaywitz et al., 2002; Simos, Fletcher, Foorman, et al., 2002). Much like adults, children with impaired reading exhibited less neural activity in left posterior regions during reading and language tasks. They also showed concomitantly greater activation in other regions of the brain when reading, such as the right hemisphere. This pattern has been interpreted as the brain's attempt to compensate for physiological deficits in the left posterior regions (Shaywitz & Shaywitz, 2005).

More intriguing, targeted educational interventions, focused on building phonological and other reading skills, can actually induce a more normalized profile of brain function in children with impaired reading acquisition (Agnew, Dorn, & Eden, 2004; Gaab, Gabrieli, Deutsch, Tallal, & Temple, 2007; Shaywitz et al., 2004; Simos, Fletcher, Bergman, et al., 2002). However, the reading itself, although improved, generally does not approach age-referenced proficiency in terms of fluency and comprehension.

All in all, the neuroimaging studies seem tell a coherent story, consistent with the basic premise of a dysfunctional cognitive module, present in children and adults alike, that impairs reading acquisition. This module is apparently responsive to repair by evidence-based training therapies. Moreover, the neuroimaging studies seem to converge with genetic studies that, as described above, indicate that the candidate genes are expressed in brain regions that are functionally associated with reading. The emerging picture appears to outline a direct pathway from gene to brain, cognition, behavior, and even to repairing the defective module.

Yet the picture is actually more complex, as with most phenomena of this sort. As described above, candidate genes that have been repeatedly linked to dyslexia show widespread expression throughout the brain, not only in areas most closely linked to reading. Moreover, genes linked to reading may be equally linked to math and language, raising the possibility of "generalist genes." Although evidence-based therapies apparently normalize brain function, the children's functional reading nonetheless remains below par on most dimensions even though brain function has improved. This complexity is commensurate with the complexity of the clinical phenomena being studied and is in keeping with a developmental process. Understanding learning problems, therefore, will require integration of this genetic and neuroscientific literature with perspectives provided by developmental science.

Much of what we know about development comes not only from studies of children, but also from careful observation of, and experimentation on, behavioral development in other species. The basic developmental *processes* are relatively similar not only across human skills or capacities but also across species. Processes observed in a variety of animal studies can be directly relevant to our understanding of developmental disorders, in general, and of learning disorders more specifically. With this in mind, we detour briefly from our discussion of learning disabilities per se to the developmental perspective itself. Some of this discussion may initially seem irrelevant to learning disorders. However, armed with principles and concepts derived from this work, we will shortly return to children with learning disorders.

PROCESSES OF BEHAVIORAL DEVELOPMENT: ANIMAL STUDIES

In 1973 the Nobel prize in physiology or medicine was awarded to three behavioral scientists, a remarkable achievement in an arena that is regularly dominated by the basic medical sciences. The awardees were ethologists Konrad Lorenz, Nikolaas Tinbergen, and Karl von Frisch, who achieved the honor for challenging prevailing assumptions about the instinctive nature of behavior and its development. Through careful observation and analysis, they demonstrated that behaviors that appear instinctive actually depend on external triggers, to which the young animal is sensitive during "critical periods" of development.

In the most famous demonstration, Lorenz raised newborn ducklings so that during the first hours of life, as they began to move independently, they did not see their mother but only the scientist himself. These ducklings then followed Lorenz slavishly, just as if he were their mother. A photograph of little ducklings following an elderly German professor now adorns many introductory psychology texts. Lorenz proved that ducklings are not born with an instinct to follow their mother; rather, they follow the first large animate object they see, which, in the natural world, is almost universally the mother duck. The work of Lorenz and the other ethologists revolutionized our understanding not only of animal behavior but also of human behavioral development and ultimately human nature itself.

In the United States students of animal behavior such as T. C. Schneirla, Daniel Lehrman, and Frank Beach challenged the European ethologists for not going far enough. The Europeans had concluded that innate behavioral patterns needed only to be *released* by specific experiential triggers. The Americans, through careful laboratory experimentation, analyzed the well-choreographed interplay between physiological mechanisms such as neural and hormonal responses, experience, and behavioral patterns. This line of work demonstrated a developmental principle with profound implications for our appreciation of human behavior: *Behavioral patterns that appear inborn and genetically preprogrammed can be a function of complex interactions between the developing organism and its physical and social environment.* Because many of these environmental stimuli are so universal or all-encompassing, the behaviors appear to be innate. This insight echoes Piaget's assertion that heredity presupposes *"an action of the environment and a reaction of the organism"* (Piaget, 1963, p. 18). Because of the complexity of organism–environment interactions, variations in either biological or environmental characteristics can cause functions to develop in a suboptimal fashion. To the extent that these become maladaptive, they may come to be classified as disorders or disabilities.

The fundamental message of these studies is that intuitive assumptions about the causes and development of behavior must constantly be challenged and questioned. This challenge should also apply to our thinking about learning disorders. Any tidy scenario in which a gene *causes* a difference in brain structure, which in turn *causes* a functional disability involving a specific skill or skills (e.g., reading or math), must be viewed with caution.

This developmental tradition is exemplified by the work of three scientists: Gilbert Gottlieb, Mark Johnson, and Annette Karmiloff-Smith. Although each approaches the processes of behavioral development differently, their insights are germane to learning disorders. Gottlieb worked primarily in animal behavior and extracted principles that extend to human development; Johnson, who studies infants, and Karmiloff-Smith, who studies children with genetic disorders, are clearly influenced by Gottlieb as well as by Piagetian traditions. Together, they provide a way of thinking about children with developmental differences, such as learning problems, that is different from the prevailing view.

Gilbert Gottlieb: Relational Causality

Gilbert Gottlieb was a seminal theorist in the world of developmental behavioral science. Trained as a comparative psychologist, he drew on experimental studies of animal behavioral development to understand processes of human development and especially developmental psychopathology. Developmental processes can be easier to discern in animals, in part because the behavioral repertoire is simpler and more stereotyped, in part because experiments are possible that could not be implemented with children for ethical or practical reasons, and in part because the developmental process is telescoped in animals with shorter lifespans. A bird or rodent can be observed from the prenatal period through sexual maturation and adulthood within a relatively brief human time frame. Principles gleaned from these studies provide insights into processes of human behavioral development, sometimes challenging assumptions that seem intuitively obvious. Although it is rare that mechanisms in animal behavior can be applied directly to human behavior, these studies can stimulate novel hypotheses about human behavioral development (Gottlieb & Lickliter, 2004).

The biological concept of *epigenesis* is central to Gottlieb's thinking. Epigenesis is the developmental process whereby each successive stage of development builds on foundations laid down by preceding stages. Thus, if Gene A is statistically associated with Behavior B in a population, the gene does not necessarily lead directly to the behavior. Rather, Gene A is proximally associated with Behavior B1, which in turn gives rise to B2, which gives rise to B3, and so forth, until the adult phenotypic behavioral profile is attained. The modern concept of epigenesis stands in contrast to earlier *preformist* notions, according to which development is simply the maturation of a preformed entity. Gottlieb and Halpern (2002) criticized a persistent preformist bias in the study of human behavior genetics. They contrasted *"predetermined* epigenesis" with what they called *"probabilistic* epigenesis." In predetermined epigenesis each developmental stage emerges from the prior one, unfolding in a linear programmed fashion as if hardwired. Thus, in our highly ingrained and intuitive understanding of child development, children achieve developmental "milestones" one after another, in an apparently predestined fashion along a linear trajectory. Indeed, the metaphor of a milestone suggests a well-traveled road that guides the direction of development.

In probabilistic epigenesis, in contrast, development is the product of systemic and dynamic interactions among genes, brain, and experience. Although functional change over time may appear to unfold in a predetermined way, it is in fact *activity-dependent*, emerging from and fundamentally dependent upon these interactions. A key concept for our discussion is the notion that subtle biases in the system will influence the nature of a being's experience, resulting in the emergence of more specific and complex behavioral patterns. Significantly, these various levels of function—genetic, neurobiological, hormonal, experiential—are "coactive": That is, they are so interdependent that they are effectively inseparable from one another, and it is therefore not possible to conclude that one follows on the other in a linear causal fashion, as illustrated in Figure 3.1. Causality, in fact, is emergent from these developmental interrelationships or systems, not a unidirectional effect of gene or even experience on behavior. Gottlieb refers to this concept as "relational causality." To understand what these concepts mean more concretely, we turn first to the avian world.

Lessons from the Birds

The avian world offers elegant examples of the developmental processes described above. A simple example of probabilistic epigenesis can be seen in the barnyard chicken's characteristic pecking at the earth for worms and grubs. This chicken behavior is so universal that the pecking seems innate, genetically programmed to appear shortly after hatching. In an ingenious experiment, however, Wallman (1979) housed newly hatched chicks individually inside plain white cardboard cylinders (actually, ice cream containers) for the first few days of life. Just after they had hatched, he placed white taffeta booties on half the chicks so that they could walk but could not see their toes; the rest went barefoot as chickens normally do. After 2 days, both groups were presented with mealworms, standard chicken fare. Remarkably, the chicks shod in booties were baffled by the worms; many initially ran away, and few ate them. The chicks that had seen their toes, however, as if by instinct, immediately began pecking at the worms. Similar effects were seen when the toes were painted black.

So, it turned out that pecking at worms is not as instinctive for chickens as it appears, but requires early visual experience to stimulate the behavior. Visual exposure to a stimulus as minimal (but evolutionarily guaranteed to be there) as their own toes, was sufficient to enable pecking behavior, essential to their survival, to emerge. Even the chicks that had worn the booties soon began to peck at the worms once the booties were removed. Although only minimal visual experience is needed to prime the behavior, *some* visual experience is necessary. The *probability* that a newly hatched chick will have sufficient visual experience, even if that experience is only of its own toes, is so exceedingly high, and the survival value of feeding is so great, that worm pecking is

BIDIRECTIONAL INFLUENCES

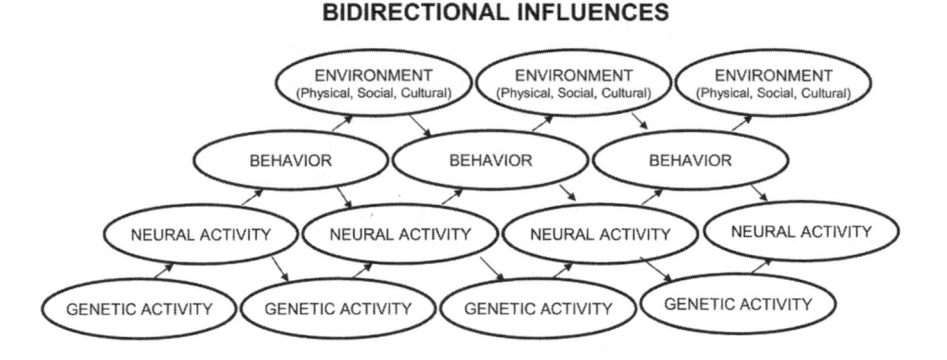

FIGURE 3.1. The various roles that experience plays during the course of anatomical, physiological, behavioral, and psychological development. Based on Gottlieb (1992).

virtually universal. Since most chickens are not reared in ice cream containers wearing taffeta booties, this learning process—the probabilistic epigenesis—is typically masked, and the behavior appears instinctive.

Perhaps more directly relevant to learning disorders is the elegant story of vocal learning in songbirds, detailed over decades by Fernando Nottebohm and his students. Bird song is a complex and highly developed skill that serves a crucial adaptive social function, attracting females to mate and thus procreate the species. Male songbirds, like children learning language, exhibit a lengthy period of song development, starting with a babbling-like vocalization, called "pre-song," followed by a more variable but recognizable song, called "plastic song," and finally the stable adult song (Nottebohm, 2005). For individual birds, song development does not unfold in a stereotyped fashion but can be idiosyncratic, as if each bird needed to solve the problem for himself (Liu, Gardner, & Nottebohm, 2004). Indeed, these birds even develop neighborhood dialects within the forest, mimicking the song of birds living in neighboring trees (Olofsson & Servedio, 2008), much as humans develop regional dialects. Thus, even in birds, whose behavior superficially appears stereotypical, the individual organism *constructs* behaviors as a process of interaction with expectable experience, and subtle variations emerge as a result of these interactions.

The developmental neurobiological mechanisms underlying the acquisition of bird song, which are available to experimental analysis, provide perspective on the very important neurobiological mechanisms associated with human language acquisition. The neuroanatomy of the brain circuits supporting song has been exquisitely described (Notte-bohm, 2005). An anterior circuit in the forebrain is primarily involved in song acquisition, and a posterior circuit is needed for both acquisition and production. Some species even exhibit lateralization, with song con-trolled primarily by one hemisphere, similar to humans in whom the left hemisphere is typically dominant for speech (Nottebohm, 1971).

Male zebra finches display two kinds of song: *directed* song, in which the song is directed to a female as part of a courting ritual, accompanied by a stylized dance; and *undirected* song, in which males sing in the presence of other males or alone. Undirected song is thought to be the vehicle for learning the song. In an article aptly entitled, "For Whom the Bird Sings," Jarvis and colleagues (Jarvis, Scharff, Gross-man, Ramos, & Nottebohm, 1998) reported that gene expression in the anterior circuit depends on the social context. Recall that gene expres-sion is the process by which information encoded in the DNA is trans-lated into a physiological function of the cell. Genes are expressed not only during embryological development, but can be turned off and on throughout the lifespan. When a male zebra finch sings in the presence of other males, the *ZENK* gene, important for learning, is expressed at much higher levels than when the bird directs his song to a female that he is courting. The salience of the *social context* is underscored by the fact that this phenomenon can occur even in deafened birds, indicat-ing that gene expression is not triggered simply by auditory stimulation but by social proximity. This social responsiveness, moreover, is medi-ated by dopamine, a neurotransmitter that is abundant in the anterior "learning" brain circuit (Sasaki, Sotnikova, Gainetdinov, & Jarvis, 2006). Some sensory aspect of social contact presumably stimulates relevant neurons to fire, thereby modifying dopamine levels, which in turn influence expression of the *ZENK* gene that presumably facilitates learning.

The working hypothesis here is that undirected singing, and the neu-rochemical changes associated with it, maintains the song in good work-ing order for the less frequent occasions when it is needed for directed singing—that is, when the male bird is courting a female, essential for reproduction. The increased expression of *ZENK* facilitates learning, stimulated by social contact with other males, who themselves similarly benefit from the social contact in terms of song acquisition and mainte-nance.

These observations of developmental processes in birds, it turns out, have surprising application to humans. Goldstein, King, and West (2003) drew on songbird studies to reexamine prevailing assumptions about infant speech learning. The dominant model was that infants learned speech primarily through imitation as the motor articulators matured sufficiently to support it. Inspired by the bird model, however, Goldstein and his colleagues wondered whether infant speech acquisition might also depend on social feedback. In their experiment, 8-month-old infants and their mothers visited the laboratory, and the mothers were instructed to provide *social* feedback (smiling, moving closer to the infant, touching), either contingent on the child's speech production or noncontingently, when instructed by the experimenter to respond. In fact, the children who received contingent social responding not only demonstrated an increase in the number of speech sounds, but their speech was also more advanced phonologically than their baseline performance. Infant babbling, parallel to song learning in birds, both regulates and is regulated by social interaction. Here again, developmentally motivated research illustrates how the construction by the child (or bird) of a specific function depends on the availability of expectable experiences, some of which may not appear to have a direct (modular) connection with the specific skill. The study also raises intriguing questions about how deviations in the system (e.g., maternal depression, insensitivity of child to social stimuli) could modify the course of speech and language development.

The key point is that a molecular function in the brain, namely, gene expression, is *embedded in a system that is not confined to the brain or even to the individual bird or child.* This system anticipates and depends on a particular kind of social experience that modulates gene expression in ways that are fundamentally advantageous for the species—again, probabilistic epigenesis. Thus, Jarvis and colleagues (1998) conclude that "if molecular biology is to achieve its full impact on the understanding of brain function, it will have to devote as much scrutiny to the behaviors it tries to explain as to the molecules that are involved" (p. 784). As Gottlieb and Halpern (2002) argued, boundaries among genes, brain, experience, and behavior become indistinct within a developing system. In humans, with their complex and diverse lives, different kinds of experiences will occur with different probabilities, and these experiences can have a material influence on processes of brain development.

Human Psychopathology: The 5-HTT Gene

The basic developmental principle described for birds—that is, that gene expression depends on experience—has wide application in understanding behavioral development, including human behavioral development. Conceptual innovations derived from comparative psychology, neuroscience, and genetics are bearing fruit in cutting-edge discoveries in developmental psychopathology.

The unfolding story of the *5-HTT* gene provides an excellent model for understanding these potential gene–environment interactions. This gene encodes for the transport of serotonin, a neurotransmitter that is crucial for mood regulation. An important region of this gene is present in humans as either a long or a short version (allele). Individuals who carry two copies of the short version (homozygous) are at increased risk for depression and other mood disorders (Collier et al., 1996). But this association is by no means consistent (Veenstra-VanderWeele, Anderson, & Cook, 2000); only some people who carry this risk gene develop a mood disorder. This important phenomenon has been analyzed both experimentally and epidemiologically.

Since the rhesus monkey carries a gene analogous to the human *5-HTT*, its role in behavioral development has been addressed experimentally in the laboratory, building on the important but disturbing work of Harry Harlow. After World War II, the plight of orphaned children was a great social concern, stimulating developmental psychologists to study the foundations of infant attachment. In the laboratory, Harry Harlow studied the behavior of infant monkeys reared without their mothers. Again, burned into our consciousnesses from introductory psychology textbooks are the poignant photographs of baby monkeys clinging to surrogate mothers made of wire and toweling and equipped with a mechanical teat, documenting the intense drive of the infant primate for social contact with its mother.

Using the Harlow paradigm, researchers (Champoux et al., 2002) raised a group of monkeys with peers only, without access to the parent, a highly stressful condition for baby monkeys. These monkeys were compared with typically reared animals. Infants that carried the risk allele were more emotionally reactive than those that did not, but significantly, only if they had been reared in the high-stress condition. Moreover, among peer-reared animals, those who carried the risk allele had lower serotonin concentrations than did those that did not, but there was no such association of neurotransmitter levels with the allele for normally reared animals. Monkeys raised by their parents were apparently *protected* from the potential risk conferred by the gene, demonstrable not only behaviorally but also neurochemically.

Human epidemiological data show a similar pattern. The Dunedin Multidisciplinary Health and Development Study is a large population-based study in New Zealand. It presented a unique opportunity to examine these developmental processes through naturalistic observation (Caspi et al., 2003). Over 1,000 children were followed regularly from birth to young adulthood. Young adults who had been maltreated as children were more vulnerable to depression if they carried the *5-HTT* risk allele; those who did not carry the allele were much less likely to become depressed, even if maltreated. Conversely, like the monkeys, children who had not experienced maltreatment showed no correlation between the risk allele and depression (Figure 3.2).

When the Dunedin children reached age 26, the researchers asked them about stressful life events in the previous 5 years. Although people who did and did not carry the risk allele were equally likely to experience stressful events, those who were homozygous for the risk allele (i.e., they carried two rather than one copy) were much more likely to become depressed than those without the risk allele if they experienced such events. The response was dose dependent, moreover; the more events they experienced, the more severe their symptoms. Thus, the risk allele increases the likelihood of a depressive disorder, but only if the developing child is exposed to extreme stress; by the same token, children who

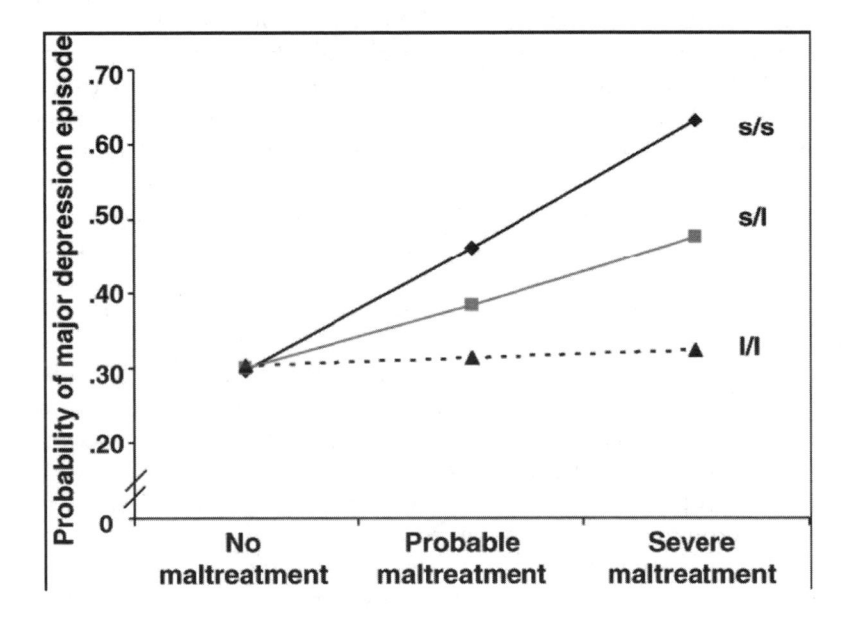

FIGURE 3.2. Results of regression analysis estimating the association between childhood maltreatment (between the ages of 3 and 11 years) and adult depression (ages 18–26), as a function of the *5-HTT* genotype. The short allele (*s*) confers higher risk than the long (*l*) allele. The *s/s* group is homozygous for the short allele; the *s/l* group is heterozygous; and the *l/l* group is homozygous for the long allele. Early maltreatment increases risk for major depression in the *s/s* and *s/l* groups but not the *l/l* group. From Caspi, A., et al. (2003). Influence of life stress on depression: Moderation by a polymorphism in the 5-HTT gene. *Science, 301,* 386–389. Copyright by the Association for the Advancement of Science. Reprinted by permission.

experience stress are less vulnerable to its effects if they do not carry the risk allele.

The actual statistics, however, emphasize the *probabilistic* nature of these epigenetic processes. Among people who had experienced four or more stressful life events, 33% of those homozygous for the risk allele had become depressed, compared with only 17% of those who were not; but 10% of those with neither the risk allele nor stressful events experienced major depression. In other words, two-thirds of those at high risk (both genetically and stress-related) had not yet experienced a depressive episode, and 10% of those at low risk (both genetically and stress-related) did experience such an episode. Thus, the end state reflects multiple interacting risk and protective factors; psychopathology is by no means inevitable, even for those at high environmental and genetic risk. These fascinating clinical studies are entirely consonant with Gottlieb's notions of relational causality and probabilistic epigenesis, concepts "hatched" from experiments with other species.

Mark Johnson: Interactive Specialization

Mark Johnson has applied the above developmental ideas to the study of human infants, focusing primarily on face processing. Like Gottlieb, Johnson is skeptical of developmental models that presuppose innate faculties as direct precursors of the more modular structure of adult cognition (Johnson, 2003). Drawing on the notion of probabilistic epigenesis, Johnson (2000) argues that the ontogeny of the neural substrates for behavioral and cognitive function is highly dynamic and experience dependent. According to his "interactive specialization" model, cognition and affect develop as a result of the specialization of multiple coactive pathways. Development depends on the continual activity of these pathways, which serve importantly to construct and establish interregional interactions that are essential to support cognitive and affective functioning. Although these capacities are not initially organized in a modular fashion, developmental processes ultimately result in the stabler adult modular organization. Thus, functional development is a process of organization and construction of interregional interactions rather than the "maturation" of a specific region (Johnson, 2001). Functions, moreover, do not reside in any particular structure but in distributed functional networks that, over time, become self-organized, streamlined, and, with repeated experience, specialized for a particular capacity. Whereas an execution of a particular function might recruit brain activity from more extensive regions in a young child, over time and as a function of development, the adult organization emerges, with areas of activation that are more efficient and anatomically restricted. Adult-type associations between structure and function thus evolve as a function of development, nourished by activity and experience. The interactive specialization concept may seem abstract, but it is actually familiar from everyday life, albeit in very different contexts.

A Real-World Example of Interactive Specialization

Consider two young and relatively inexperienced college students who decide to start a business. Joe enjoys playing with computers and has an idea for a software application he thinks will sell. His friend Don has taken a few business courses, and so they team up. At first they do some informal research, surf the Web, and refine their ideas in late-night dorm conversations. Then, with a little financial support from their parents, they enlist others—a finance consultant, a software engineer. For the first few years they work out of a garage and are pretty much on their own, developing the software, devising a business plan, figuring out marketing strategies, and setting up a website. Working side by side in the garage, they interact constantly, and both are involved to some extent in all the tasks and issues that arise.

Here is where interactive specialization enters the picture. In the early years, Joe and Don are both intensely involved in the technical and business development sides of the enterprise, though each tends to be more assertive in his own area of interest and competence. Because the business is small and new, both function as a jack-of-all-trades. As the business grows, however, they increasingly build on their initial talents and skills and become more specialized. Joe becomes deeply involved with product development, spending time testing out different options. Meanwhile, Don focuses on implementing the business plan. Soon, Joe is spending most of his time working with the software engineer on perfecting the product, while Don works with the financial analyst to access venture capital and organize the business systems. As the enterprise begins to take off, each hires more expert staff in his area, as well as more support staff.

By now, the business has moved to rented office space, and each partner has his own administrative assistant. Increasingly, Joe loses touch with the business side and Don with the technical side, as they become more specialized within their own departments and it makes less sense for them to spend time working on aspects of the business in which they do not have expertise. Instead of relying on themselves to know the whole business, they need to formalize an organizational structure so that the technical and business sides are not only effective in executing their own functions, but communicate and complement one another as well.

In the process of growing to achieve its goal of developing and marketing software, the company has acquired a complex organizational structure that encompasses two fundamental developmental processes: *specialization* and *integration*. Specialization involves the commitment of a particular structural component to a particular function; integration involves the coordination of component specialized functions in the service of a more complex organismic goals. The structural organization emerged from the process of performing a goal-directed function, and the function likewise emerged from the organization. Like the chicken and the egg, it would be hard to claim that one causal direction takes precedence over the other.

After 3 years the business employs 100 people organized into four departments, some reporting ultimately to Joe and some to Don. Happily for Joe and Don, 5 years later, the business has grown to 1,800 employees, and they sell it for $20 million. The company now functions independently, with new leadership and without Joe and Don, who have retired to villas in Tuscany and are contemplating their next venture.

According to the interactive specialization model, complex brain functions develop like a start-up company. The infant brain has multiple potential pathways, whose functional specialization emerges from subtle intrinsic differences in their initial connectivity (i.e., what connects most efficiently to what), the density of synaptic connections, and the speed of processing information. These subtle differences have been called "architectural constraints" (Elman, 1996). Equally important is the infant's adaptive need as an organism to accomplish basic goals (eating, sleeping, speaking, playing, loving). As the infant interacts with the environment in service of these goals, certain pathways become preferentially activated by different types of activity and experience for which they have a structural advantage. These pathways will be more routinely activated and will similarly recruit other pathways in service of the function, whereas less efficient or less appropriate pathways will be less and less involved. Recall also Nottebohm's birds, each of whom learned the species-specific song as if it were solving a new problem. Similarly, the developing child engages in a constant process of problem solving as it masters new and more complex information and skills, thereby constructing cognition, affect, and behavior.

Functional neuroimaging studies of typically developing children document the gradual shift from diffuse to focal organization in response to specific tasks (Durston et al., 2006). More importantly, neuroscientists are beginning to provide more evidence for the processes of segregation, which leads to functional specialization and integration, which are so central to the functional development of the brain and, by extension, human cognitive, affective, and behavioral functioning. Using a neuroimaging technique called "resting state functional connectivity," they can evaluate correlations among brain regions in the resting brain (i.e., when the brain is not engaged in a specific task) in order to map connectivity. In young children, connections are primarily local—that is, short-range—and between regions that are geographically close to one another. Neuronal networks that will eventually function as more specialized systems in the mature adult are more densely interconnected in younger children and even adolescents. Over time, largely stimulated by experiential transactions, the regions segregate from one another and the local connections become weaker, while connectivity among distant or distributed regions of the brain is strengthened (Fair et al., 2007, 2009), generally consistent with an interactive specialization hypothesis.

In theory, these continuing processes of segregation and integration in development make possible higher-order and more complex cognitive function. The more widely distributed and well-orchestrated networks may be needed to process larger volumes of more complex information. Furthermore, because these processes of segregation and integration occur over an extended period throughout development, they may be particularly likely candidate mechanisms underlying the subtler (high frequency–low impact) variations in cognitive functioning typically seen in children with learning disabilities. Hence, these developmental processes are highly germane to the phenomena of interest here.

The Joe and Don story also illustrates this process. As college students Joe and Don had somewhat different interests and connections, but there was also considerable overlap in their activities. As they pursued aspects of the business that were compatible with their initial interests and capabilities, however, their skills and their professional networks became increasingly distinct from one another, and they also recruited others to help them with their task as the demands grew. Equally important, the success of their enterprise depended crucially on their ability to organize and especially to *integrate* these functions.

Similarly in the brain, *pathways that have intrinsic structural advantage will be more consistently activated by a particular functional demand* (e.g., language or social interaction). Pathways that are less well suited to that function will become committed to other functions for which they are better adapted as the process of segregation advances. As these pathways are repeatedly used for particular functions, they become entrenched and "committed," resulting ultimately in the more modular functional specialization of the adult. Importantly, although the initial biases that gave rise to this specialization may still be detectable, they need no longer serve the same causal function because the network has become more routinely and automatically engaged and now functions as a coherent entity in and of itself, more than the sum of its components.

Returning once again to our business analogy, although Joe and Don have now sold the business and are off sipping Italian wine, their portraits grace the lobby of the corporate headquarters, and their initial vision continues to define the culture of the company. Nonetheless, if one wanted to institute a change at the company, one would not travel to Italy to find Joe and Don. Similarly, although footprints of earlier biases that led to the establishment of a particular functional network may be detectable, these footprints may or may not provide the optimal approach to intervention to deal with the more fully developed and entrenched functional networks of older children and adults.

And what about developmental *disorders*? How do they fit with this scheme? Suppose Joe teams up, early on, not with Don but with Scott, who is less effective than Don at holding up his end. The two set off to start a company. Joe plows ahead developing the software, but Scott, unlike Don, is out of step. He doesn't coordinate well with the finance consultant, giving him conflicting signals or failing to supply the needed figures when he says he will. Despite the quality of the software, the business falters, and Joe finds himself increasingly distracted and involved in Scott's domain, making sure that he meets deadlines and follows through with contacts. Because he is constantly monitoring Scott, Joe can pay less attention to his own area, software development, jeopardizing the success of the business. Although things continue to move forward, the company is plagued by these organizational problems and runs inefficiently, affecting the bottom line and causing considerable stress for Joe. Thus, neither specialization nor integration can occur effectively and, importantly, the effect is systemic, not confined to Scott's area of expertise. Joe ultimately brings in new leadership to handle Scott's division, after Scott agrees to take a lesser role, but the business side remains a source of concern for some time as strategies need to be developed to repair the dysfunction.

Similarly, in developmental disorders relatively minor deviations and inefficiencies at the outset can become manifest more broadly and compromise not only a specific skill most directly associated with the initial deviation, but also the efficiency of the system as a whole as it develops. Johnson and colleagues (2005) has explored these developmental processes in the context of the social brain network, primarily in relation to face processing and eye gaze in infants. Both are fundamental to successful social development. Typical adults respond to faces in characteristic ways. For example, most adults recognize faces more quickly and accurately when they are upright than when they are upside down. This preferential response suggests that in the adult, the face-processing network is finely tuned to upright faces. Since infants cannot report what they see, Johnson measures brain waves generated in response to specific stimuli (called event-related potentials, or ERPs) to find out how they perceive faces. Until about a year of age, infants respond similarly to upright and inverted faces, indicating that in the infant, face processing is incompletely differentiated. Significantly, regions that are activated by faces in adults are only partially activated by faces in the infant brain. Thus, Johnson argues, adult behavioral competence does not appear de novo because new brain regions mature and come online. Rather, relevant regions are active and available from the outset. They become more finely tuned and integrated for processing faces as a function of interactive specialization. This occurs in the matrix of daily, repeated experience looking at faces and the neural architectural constraints that support this skill.

This work on typical babies has potential relevance to autism, a developmental disorder that primarily affects social development. Johnson and colleagues (2005) have speculated that in children with autism, for whatever reason, the expected process of specialization and "tuning" of the social brain network is disordered. Whereas typical children develop well-tuned, sensitive, and acute mechanisms for processing faces and other social cues, children with autism appear to process social and nonsocial stimuli in a relatively undifferentiated manner. Ultimately, they do not develop the typical modular organization of social cognition. Retrospective analysis of home movies indicates that children do not suddenly become autistic at age 2 or 3; subtler behavioral differences can be detected very early in life (Clifford, Young, & Williamson, 2007; Palomo, Belinchon, & Ozonoff, 2006). These seemingly subtle differences may lead to increasing deviance as social cognition is constructed, albeit atypically, through interactive experience. Although this observation does not "explain" autism, it is consonant with the developmental view that the brains of affected children are not normal brains with parts intact and parts missing, but brains set on a different developmental course (Oliver et al., 2000), potentially affecting multiple aspects of their development, as is typically true for developmental disorders.

The processes involved in developmentally based disorders are therefore not localizable to discrete regions of brain; rather, they are more widespread and activity or experience dependent. Even if there are identifiable genes associated with autism spectrum disorders, their development into the full-blown syndrome may not be inevitable. By implication, if these subtle biases were detected early, it might be possible to redirect the system before the maladaptive networks became more elaborated and entrenched in the process of development, thereby mitigating some of the more severe behavioral outcomes. Understanding the relatively subtle and heterogeneous presentation of learning disorders may be profitably referenced to these systemic concepts of functional brain development.

Annette Karmiloff-Smith: A Neuroconstructivist Approach to Development

The work of Annette Karmiloff-Smith is, in many ways, most directly relevant to learning disorders. She has applied the developmental approach directly to children with developmental disabilities, specifically to groups with a known *genetic etiology*. In an article titled "Development Itself Is the Key to Understanding Developmental Disorders," Karmiloff-Smith (1998) lays out her neuroconstructivist position. She contends that the behavioral features of developmental disorders reflect the outcome of developmental processes that involve interactions among gene, child, and environment, rather than the direct expression of a gene in a specific behavioral function. Integrating Gottlieb's "probabilistic epigenesis" with developmental psychology, she argues that the contribution of genes is one of introducing initial biases into a system. Furthermore, she agrees with Johnson that the adult modular organization of cognition is the outcome of a developmental process. This position stands in contrast to assumptions that genes hold the code for specific behavioral modules, what she terms the "Swiss-Army-knife" approach.

Karmiloff-Smith (1998) argues that because of the unusually prolonged period of human development, evolution selects not for specific skills but for *particular outcomes and a strong capacity to learn*. In the same vein as Johnson, she argues that genes encode for *domain-relevant* skills, not *domain-specific* skills. What does this mean? Domain-relevant functions are those that are highly relevant to one kind of input; their repeated use in service of achieving a particular function can lead to a more "entrenched" and domain-*specific* association with a specific skill. However, these domain-relevant capacities can be recruited for other types of processing in which they may not play such a major role. Such domain-relevant functions are likely to be relatively simple and "low-level," that is, an endophenotype. An "endophenotype" is defined as a heritable trait or characteristic that is not a direct symptom of the condition under investigation but is associated with the condition. Thus, according to Karmiloff-Smith, a tiny deviation in an initial, domain-*relevant* state could give rise to much more elaborated and entrenched domain-*specific* differences in end states that are of far greater functional significance. Although the footprints of these tiny deviations may be detectable, their causal function in the mature child may be greatly diminished relative to their importance earlier in development—as with

Joe and Don, whose tangible presence in the company is reduced to a portrait hanging in the lobby.

In this scenario, elaborated functions such as language, or even components of language such as semantic meaning or grammar, are not domain-relevant functions but would be considered domain-specific. Hence they would rest on developmental processes involving subtler and low-level domain-relevant endophenotypes. The language and social environments stimulate and interact with these low-level functions nearly constantly in early development as the child strives for communication and social engagement. Since the language environment is so all-encompassing during infancy and childhood, developmental patterns can appear innate, even though they may not actually be so.

Fundamental to this developmental perspective is the concept of a *developmental cascade*, a construct that has proven especially meaningful in studies of developmental psychopathology and developmental disorders more generally (de Vries & Watson, 2008; Karmiloff-Smith, 1998; Masten et al., 2005). According to Masten and colleagues (2005), a developmental cascade occurs when "functioning in one domain of adaptive behavior spills over to influence functioning in other domains in a lasting way" (p. 735). Thus, the effects of maladaptive functioning in a domain early in development can become more pervasive or diffuse as that function affects the quality of the child's experience, amplifying its impact and ultimately becoming entrenched as a more significant disorder. This view contrasts with one that assumes developmental continuity, such that an early deficit profile will predict a fixed deficit in the same domain but not others. Masten and colleagues, for example, reported on a 20-year longitudinal study, demonstrating that externalizing behavioral problems (e.g., hyperactivity, aggression) in childhood led to subsequent worsening of academic achievement in early adolescence, which in turn led to increased internalizing symptoms (e.g., depression, anxiety) in later adolescence and young adulthood. As a result of the developmental cascade, the earlier behavioral problems spread to encompass a much broader range of functioning, extending well beyond the initial scope of the problem.

This notion of developmental cascades is germane to any developmental approach to learning disabilities; the effects of early cognitive variations, potentially genetically influenced, can become more diffusely expressed in the context of the developmental process, potentially amplifying their impact to become far more intrusive and disabling functionally. Importantly, within such a framework, the goal of intervention is not merely to remediate a defective skill but to forecast and thus prevent, contain, or arrest developmental progressions *systemically* so that they do not lead to more widespread and significant maladaptive outcomes.

DEVELOPMENTAL SCIENCE: A SUMMARY

Developmental science thus provides direction for understanding the developmental problem of learning disabilities. The guiding principles, consistent with the Piagetian principles outlined in Chapter 2, are summarized as follows:

1. Because of the indistinct boundaries between gene, brain, and environment, appearances of innateness, maturation, or predetermination should always be questioned.
2. Even minor deviations present early in life in a developing system can lead to a cascade of events resulting in more markedly divergent and entrenched developmental trajectories in the course of experiential transactions.
3. Early variations, at a genetic or neural level, are more likely to have widespread than specific or restricted effects in the developing child. Moreover, seemingly discrete functional domains (e.g., cognition, affect) shape one another mutually in the context of development.

Armed with these principles, we next examine the relatively sparse but nonetheless intriguing literature on the development of reading and language problems, and we begin to explore how this more developmental approach could help us make better sense of these disorders.

Chapter 4

A Lifespan Perspective on Learning Disabilities

LEARNING (READING)-DISABLED CHILDREN AS INFANTS: EARLY PREDICTORS

Unlike some developmental problems, which declare themselves clearly early in life, learning disorders can surface at almost any point in a child's development. Typically, they are identified when the child enters school and encounters unexpected difficulties with academic demands, although precursors can be evident before school starts. When this occurs in the developmental course, however, is variable:

- "He was a little slow to talk, and other people had trouble understanding him at first."
- "She talked on time, but she had a hard time learning to tie her shoes and button her clothing."
- "In kindergarten the teacher was concerned because he didn't learn his colors and letters."
- "She was happy until she got to first grade and the work got hard. By the end of the year she was often complaining of stomachaches in the morning."
- "The teacher was concerned in first grade because he wasn't catching on as fast as he should, so we decided to hold him back, but by the middle of second grade he was struggling again."
- "She never had any real problems until this year, in the fourth grade. Now she seems lost in a lot of her subjects, but it's worst in math."

- "We were always a little unsure of how things were going, but his grades were fine and the teachers never raised any concerns. Now, in the seventh grade, I'm seeing him struggling and discouraged, and his grades are dropping."

So, were the seeds of these problems always there, as the developmental theories just reviewed would suggest, or did the problems arise de novo at some point in the child's school career? If they were there early, why were they not apparent? How do we best understand developmental variation in the emergence of learning problems? If learning disorders are indeed developmental in origin, a lifespan perspective is required to make sense of them. But how can we study developmental precursors of learning problems if children are identified only after they begin to fail or struggle in school? To address these questions, we again turn to the scientific literature on reading, since only reading has been studied intensively. Principles derived from these studies, however, undoubtedly have broader application.

INFANT PRECURSORS OF READING PROBLEMS: INITIAL STUDIES

In an early attempt to circumvent the logical problem that learning disabilities can be identified only after a child fails in school, Hollis Scarborough (1990) devised a clever strategy. Although the genetics were only dimly understood at the time, it was common knowledge that reading problems cluster in families. Scarborough therefore recruited parents of 2-year-olds who themselves had a history of reading impairment. She then tracked the children's oral and written language development through the second grade, by which time it became clearer who had a reading disability. Three groups of children emerged: children of reading impaired parents who themselves developed reading problems; children of reading impaired parents who learned to read normally; and children of normally reading parents who also learned to read normally. Retrospectively, then, she could characterize language function as early as 30 months of age for these three groups.

It turned out that children of reading-impaired parents who themselves went on to become reading impaired displayed subtle problems in their language competence as toddlers. Although their scores on standardized language tests were unremarkable, as is often the case in this field, detailed analysis of their spontaneous language revealed subtle differences in grammar and pronunciation, differences that persisted through the preschool period.

From a developmental perspective, these reading difficulties did not spring from the blue but could be related to earlier, albeit subtle, problems in language development. Perhaps significantly, at-risk children who did not become reading impaired were more similar in their language competence to unimpaired children of normally reading parents. Thus, an early, presumably genetically influenced, neurodevelopmental variation can become elaborated epigenetically as a more florid reading problem.

Molfese and his colleagues pushed the developmental timeline back even earlier, collecting ERPs at birth. ERPs, as detailed earlier, measure the brain's neurophysiological response to different kinds of stimuli. It is a popular strategy for infant researchers because it signals whether a child can perceive different kinds of stimuli even though he or she is not yet capable of a volitional response. Newborn speech perception, as detected by ERPs, it turned out, predicted oral language function at 3 and 5 years of age (Molfese, Betz, Molfese, & Segalowitz, 1988; Molfese & Molfese, 1997) and ultimately single-word reading at 8 years of age (Molfese, 2000). These studies provided the first evidence of an endophenotype—a variation in neural function related specifically to speech perception and present from birth—that could be a developmental precursor of later reading problems. The model driving these studies, however, is still essentially *modular*: A presumed genetic risk codes for an initial difference in the language system that then affects the development of phonological awareness and ultimately reading.

The Jyväskylä Longitudinal Study of Dyslexia

The most comprehensive study of the precursors of reading is the Jyväskylä Longitudinal Study of Dyslexia (Lyytinen et al., 2001), an ambitious, population-based study from Finland that tracked children at family risk for reading impairment and a comparison group of children without known risk from birth through 9 years of age. The researchers initially surveyed all expectant families in the Finnish city of Jyväskylä and surrounding communities between 1993 and 1996, more than 8,000 in all. They eventually identified 410 parents with suspected dyslexia who were willing to participate in an individual assessment. Those who met the stringent criteria for the study (dyslexia in a parent and a close relative) were recruited. As in the Scarborough and Molfese studies, the primary hypothesis was that a speech perception deficit present at birth gives rise to dyslexia later in life. This study, however, also evaluated coexisting developmental issues, such as self-regulation, as well as infant motor development, temperament, and environmental factors that could influence the emergence of a reading problem, thereby allowing for a more complex developmental model.

At school age, a child's risk for reading difficulty, not surprisingly, differed depending on whether the parent had reading impairment. Children in the "at-risk" group were three times as likely be poor readers (Puolakanaho et al., 2007), and even adequate readers from that group were less advanced than those in the control group. As predicted, newborns in the at-risk group responded differently to speech sounds by ERP, and by 6 months, the groups displayed subtle but reliable differences in their ability to categorize speech sounds (Guttorm et al., 2005). Equally interesting, the reading-disabled parents of children in these two groups themselves perceived speech sounds differently (Lyytinen et al., 2004). By 2½ years of age, differences in receptive language skills were apparent.

Some of the findings, however, were less predictable. For example, the ERP difference was more prominent in the *right* hemisphere of the brain than in the language-dominant left hemisphere (Leppanen et al., 2002), suggesting not a defect in one part of the brain but a broader functional reorganization of the whole brain. These findings echo those of the Shaywitz group (Chapter 3), but suggest that the reorganization may not be a response to a single defective cognitive module; rather, some bias may be present early in life. If so, it would not be surprising that the cognitive issues these children display are not confined to a specific skill area, but can be more diverse.

Clinically, children in the at-risk group who talked late continued to exhibit language delays, whereas children in the control group who talked late were likely to catch up. Language competence predicted reading at school entry, but only for the children at familial risk.

A fascinating twist emerged, however, when the researchers considered motor development (Viholainen, Ahonen, Cantell, Lyytinen, & Lyytinen, 2002; Viholainen et al., 2006). At-risk children whose motor development was delayed during the first year of life had more limited vocabularies and shorter sentences at both 18 and 24 months and poorer language competence at 3 and 5 years of age. At age 7 the at-risk children with slow motor development read more poorly than children in the control group, even children in the control group with slow motor development. Children in the genetically at-risk group with good motor development, however, read as well as children in the control group! None of these groups differed in general cognitive ability or attentional competence. Thus, the poorer language and reading skills of the children at family risk appear to be referable almost entirely to the subgroup with slow motor development!

Why should this subgroup be at such great risk? And why did children with delayed motor development read normally if they had no family history of reading problems? One possibility is that the genetic mechanism that leads to impaired reading also affects motor development. If so, delayed motor development may be a marker for that mechanism. The researchers, however, proposed another potential pathway that could help to elaborate a developmental system in ways suggested in the previous chapter. They cite developmental psychology research that shows how independent locomotion dramatically alters the child's social, cognitive, and emotional environment (Campos et al., 2000). A crawling baby has a more restricted visual range in terms of both objects and people than a walking child. As the child learns to walk and move about more freely, opportunities for interaction increase substantially; interest in distant objects, in particular, increases, stimulating language development as well as joint attention and referential gestures. This developmental perspective raises the possibility that a genetically influenced risk (e.g., affecting auditory processing, motor development) can become amplified systemically through the child's interaction with the environment—a developmental cascade. In the spirit of Gottlieb's probabilistic epigenesis, Johnson's interactive specialization, and even Nottebohm's finches, cognitive and behavioral development is embedded in a system and not a simple linear path from gene to brain to behavior.

NONLINGUISTIC AUDITORY PROCESSING
AND LANGUAGE DEVELOPMENT

Variation in speech perception, detectable as early as birth, can predict later reading and language competence. Yet even as simple a function as perception of a speech sound may itself depend on an even more fundamental element of auditory perceptual processing. In the mid-1970s, Tallal and Piercy (1975) reported that children with language impairment have difficulty accurately identifying not only speech sounds but also rapidly occurring nonlinguistic tones. The experimental paradigm is simple: Two tones of different pitch (e.g., low–low, low–high) are presented in sequence and the child presses a button to indicate whether the tones are the same or different. The tone pairs are separated by varying intervals (ranging from 10 to 250 milliseconds). At very brief intervals (70 milliseconds), children with language impairment had greater difficulty perceiving the tones. Because speech perception and discrimination depend on the ability to perceive fast transitions in the speech signal, Tallal argued, this very basic "low level" difference may evolve to become manifest in speech perception and ultimately language development. Taking the hypothesis one step further, she demonstrated that children with dyslexia had difficulty discriminating rapidly presented tones, suggesting that perhaps this mechanism contributes to reading problems as well (Tallal, 1980).

These findings have provoked considerable, often vehement, debate. Tallal and her colleagues have developed interventions to train the brain to process fast transitions in the speech stream, which she and her colleagues claim can lead to improved language competence and possibly even improved reading (Scientific Learning, 2005; Tallal et al,, 1996). Others have argued strenuously against her position, stressing that reading, in particular, depends on an ability to segment sounds at a phonological level (e.g., *cat* = /k/ + /at/), that the putative defect in auditory processing is not well proven, and that functionally it is simply irrelevant (Mody, Studdert-Kennedy, & Brady, 1997).

This dispute has been clarified somewhat by functional brain imaging studies. As it turns out, the same regions of the auditory cortex that process speech sounds also process the temporal changes in these nonspeech sounds (Zaehle, Wustenberg, Meyer, & Jancke, 2004). Since these functions essentially share the same "real estate" in the brain, it is entirely plausible that dysfunction in that region could affect perception of both types of auditory stimuli. Whether one bears a causal relation to the other in a developmental sense, however, is less clear and perhaps not even meaningful.

One obvious question, however, is whether infants at familial risk for language and reading problems also process fast transitions of nonspeech auditory stimuli differently. In fact, at 6 months of age infants with a family history of language learning impairment showed a poorer ERP response to rapidly presented nonlinguistic auditory stimuli (Benasich et al., 2006). Moreover, the infant's response to fast transitions, like the response to speech sounds, predicted language competence at 3 years. In Karmiloff-Smith's terms, these very subtle variations can be understood as *domain-relevant* features that become elaborated in the context of a developing system to more complex, *domain-specific* outcomes such as oral language and reading. Moreover, the same physiologically affected region of cortex could give rise to problems in multiple, more elaborated, functions. Thus, a genetic variant is likely to be associated with multiple domain-relevant neural variations. And the same genetic variant is likely to be expressed in multiple regions of the brain, as the brain is being constructed and also in adulthood. Reading may be the most prominent of these because it carries such a high social premium for today's children, but it is unlikely to be unique.

DEVELOPMENT OF LEARNING DISABILITIES

How does this research help us to understand learning problems? First, the infant studies provide convincing evidence that very early and often *subtle* biases in the system can become elaborated in the context of development, just as Gottlieb, Johnson, and Karmiloff-Smith suggest. Although the particular studies focus on language and reading, such biases are likely to occur in a variety of combinations, potentially resulting in multiple interacting pathways that could become troublesome in the school context. The outcome is further complicated by the systemic interactions that can either promote or diminish the impact of these underlying differences.

Some of the findings also lend support to a more systemic developmental approach. For example, in the Jyväskylä study, newborn ERPs detected differences in speech perception between children with or without a family history of dyslexia. However, the difference did not appear primarily in the language-dominant left hemisphere, as might be expected, but in the right, suggesting that a range of cognitive functions could be impacted by whatever the variation might be. Moreover, among the children in the at-risk group, only those with delayed motor development exhibited later language and reading problems. Again, the data from this important population-based study argue against a specific deficit and suggest a more systemic developmental process.

The intriguing role of the motor system invokes Gottlieb's concept of relational causality. Children do not develop by a program of maturational unfolding, nor is their development purely "shaped" like a Skinnerian pigeon. Rather, developmental science teaches that development is a complex transactional process. The Finnish researchers acknowledge this possibility, suggesting that a child whose motor development is advanced may be better able to *seek out* opportunities for language and communicative development—experience that can then feed back into the system. Environmental affordances could thus amplify the impact of a relatively subtle, genetically influenced, risk.

If this all sounds complex and confusing, it should! But as the vignettes at the beginning of this chapter reflect, the real-life phenomenology of children with learning problems is also complex and confusing, far more complex than much of the research and clinical literature admits. The perplexing heterogeneity of presentation by children with learning problems, however, can make far more sense in a systemic developmental framework.

So how do children diagnosed with learning disorders actually fare as they become adults? When a child encounters learning problems in school, the parents may lie awake at night with nagging worries. They may fear that the child will become so discouraged by persistent struggles and failures that he or she will be crippled by psychological problems. They wonder whether and how the child will achieve the basic tasks of adulthood, being productive and satisfied at work, earning a good living, and having successful and rewarding friendships and family relationships. For most families, these outcomes are the bottom line, much more important than how well the child can actually read or compute. In 21st-century America, and in a competitive global economy, the educational bar is constantly being raised. Children must succeed at competency examinations to graduate from high school, and a college education is increasingly mandatory for a job that pays a good wage. Parents understandably may fear the worst when these goals appear to be in jeopardy. Is the anxiety justified, or is the reality more reassuring? Although research on long-term adult outcomes is sparse, consistent themes emerge. These themes, which are reviewed in the balance of this chapter, potentially inform the ways in which we understand and deal with children who "have" learning disorders and how we counsel their families.

WHEN LEARNING-DISABLED CHILDREN GROW UP

The Early Research on Long-Term Outcomes

The first comprehensive study of adult outcomes of learning-disabled children was conducted by Otfried Spreen in Vancouver, British Columbia. In a book entitled *Learning Disabled Children Growing Up,* Spreen (1988) described in great detail the lives of 255 young adults who had been evaluated for a learning disability when they were between 8 and 12 years of age. He evaluated these children at age 18 and then again at 25. Spreen found that the learning problems persisted to some degree in adulthood. Significantly, adjustment problems seemed to peak in adolescence and then decline. This developmental pattern would be replicated in other studies on adult outcomes.

Spreen painted a bleak picture. As adults, the learning-disabled individuals fared less well than their typically developing peers on nearly every life dimension: employment, income, physical and mental health, independent living, and social relationships. As young adults, a substantial number were living in supervised housing or with their parents. To quote Spreen, "Not only do these youngsters suffer through a miserable and usually shortened school career, live a discouraging social life, full of disappointments and failures, they also have fewer chances for adequate employment and advanced training" (p. 133).

The children in this study, however, were not representative of the universe of children with learning disorders. Although Spreen had excluded children with low IQ or significant emotional disturbance, approximately two-thirds of his participants had some kind of neurological impairment, such as epilepsy, accompanying the learning problems, and these more impaired children accounted for the poorer outcomes. Moreover, the children were first evaluated between 1966 and 1972, when there was little support for, or understanding of, children with learning problems, and the impact of the learning problems on life outcomes would presumably have been exacerbated.

Several years later, Maggie Bruck (1985) described a group of young adults from predominantly middle-class backgrounds in Montreal who had also been referred for diagnosis as children. Unlike Spreen, however, she excluded neurologically impaired children from the study. Her conclusions were very different. Although the learning issues persisted, they were by no means disabling in terms of fundamental life outcomes, work and family, when these individuals were compared to their unaffected siblings. As young adults, they had generally managed their learning issues well and were leading productive and satisfying lives despite their academic troubles as children. The absence of neurological impairment and their socioeconomic advantage presumably worked in their favor.

These early studies provided the first answers to questions at the heart of our concerns about learning disorders. Although the studies differed significantly in their methods and conclusions, both treated the early learning disorder and the adult outcome as a straightforward cause-and-effect relationship: learning disorder as cause, adult outcome as effect.

The next generation of researchers adopted a more nuanced developmental perspective, recognizing that the *context* within which a learning problem occurs—including factors internal to the child, such as temperament, and factors external to the child, such as family relationships—can also shape adult outcome. A child with a particular cognitive profile in one context can have a poor outcome as an adult, whereas a child in another context with a very similar profile can do quite well. In a developmental framework, in which the focus is broadly on the child rather than narrowly on the skill, *context is fundamental.* Its role in shaping the developmental course of learning disorders cannot be overemphasized.

Risk and Resilience in Children with Learning Disorders

Within this more developmental framework, researchers shifted their focus to factors that could *increase risk* or *promote resilience* for children with learning problems. The risk and resilience model, borrowed from developmental psychopathology research (Garmezy, Garmezy, & Rutter, 1983), was most clearly articulated in relation to learning-disabled children by Morrison and Cosden (1997). For both the child and the family, they suggested, a learning disorder constitutes a developmental *risk*. The *significance and meaning* of this risk, however, depends to a great extent on contextual factors (within the child, within the family, within the community), which can themselves carry risk or, equally important, protect the child from adverse outcomes. Thus, for example, a child who is at familial risk for anxiety or depression may have greater difficulty coping with the effects of a learning disorder than a child who is more resilient affectively. Or a child from an immigrant family who does not have a parent who is able to advocate on his or her behalf can have greater difficulty coping with a learning disorder than will a child from a well-acculturated middle-class family with a strong parent advocate. At the same time, a child who has well-developed social skills and a supportive school environment may cope better with a learning disorder. In the long run, these risk and protective factors, many of which can be substantially influenced by the school and family, often have a far more potent impact on adult outcome and adjustment than the learning disorder itself.

Morrison and Cosden (1997) also noted the importance of the "fit" of the individual with the environment. The ecocultural system (Keogh & Weisner, 1993), they point out, can define the meaning of the learning disorder, and this meaning can have powerful effects on long-term outcome. As with many childhood problems, family context can be especially important. Parental acceptance of the learning problem and acknowledgment of the child's strengths, be they in or out of school, can moderate the adverse impact of in-school stress. Whereas parental understanding can be protective, parental disappointment and rigidity about expectations can increase long-term psychosocial risk. Schools can also play a role. Children whose families become embroiled in contentious interactions with schools experience more stress, with adverse developmental consequences.

Importantly, within this framework of risk and resilience, Morrison and Cosden (1997) stress the crucial role that schools can play, above and beyond their didactic function, in the psychosocial development of children with learning disorders:

> To date many interventions have focused on remediation of academic problems associated with a learning disability. The diagnosis of a learning disability typically sets into motion a set of academic and school structure modifications. These interventions have a heavy emphasis on the academic needs. However, what can be done to prevent complications beyond these

academic needs? Further knowledge about risk and protective factors may help guide programs in these areas. (p. 56)

In other words, schools and families need to focus on children, not just skills.

The Children of Kauai

Although Morrison and Cosden (1997) articulated a well-developed version of a risk and resilience model for understanding learning disorders, it was Werner and Smith who first applied this approach to learning problems in their landmark epidemiological study of child development (Werner, 1993; Werner & Smith, 1992). This study tracked the development of 698 children on the Hawaiian Island of Kauai from their birth in 1955 until they were 40 years old. Epidemiological studies are particularly valuable because their findings are representative of the population at large and are not plagued by the potential bias inherent in studies that use other methods to assemble a sample. Werner and Smith followed the development of every child in the birth cohort. The remarkable length of this study, moreover, provided an opportunity to observe lifespan developmental trajectories.

Within this large epidemiological sample, 22 children were found to be learning disabled at 10 years of age (Werner, 1993). The schools had identified them for special services, and they also met a variety of clinical criteria. By today's standards, these children would be considered significantly learning impaired. As is typical in populations of children with learning disabilities, there were almost twice as many boys (14) as girls (8). Equally important, 75% came from low-income families. A control group, matched for sex, socioeconomic status, and ethnicity, was selected from the larger sample.

Because these children had been followed from birth, their early development could be examined retrospectively. Not surprisingly, the learning-disabled children had an increased history of biological risk (e.g., low birthweight, perinatal complications), and they already exhibited behavioral differences by 1 year of age. They were less affectionate and cuddly, and their mothers were viewed by social workers as more erratic and worrisome. To what extent these differences in parenting skills were a characteristic of the mothers themselves, reflected their response to a difficult baby, or both, is important to consider. This question highlights the social dynamic that can emerge in response to a child's neurodevelopmental trajectory, and, moreover, the tightly knit and potentially cascading interactions between biology and environment that can play themselves out through development. By age 2 these children were described as more awkward, distractible, and fearful. Their mothers were described either as careless and indifferent or as overprotective, again suggesting potential effects of caring for a difficult infant on the mother–child dynamic. Their physical and motor development was also more likely to have been delayed.

At age 10, the children's mean IQ was only 88, compared to 100 for the controls. Given their combined social disadvantage and developmental course, this was indeed a high-risk group. Between the ages of 10 and 18, 80% had contact with a community agency, more than any other risk group in the study and nine times higher than the controls. One of three had been referred to the Department of Education for truancy and poor school attendance, indicative of a poorly managed learning disorder; children become discouraged and disengaged from school as they encounter repeated failure. These children were twice as likely as the children in the larger cohort to have had contact with the judicial system, mostly for repetitive, impulsive behavior.

At age 18 their academic skills were still significantly delayed, particularly in reading and writing; they exhibited persistent visuomotor deficits; and they had significant psychosocial problems. They had little sense of agency: they believed that events controlled them, not that they had the power to control, or even affect, the events in their own lives. Most had only vague plans for the future, had poor social relations, and felt limited support or understanding from their parents. Only a quarter had shown improvement in their general functioning; the individuals who did show progress cited the emotional support that they had received from family members, peers, or elders who had bolstered their self-esteem. Most felt that the counselors or mental health professionals they encountered had not been particularly helpful.

What the researchers discovered when they next visited these young adults at age 32 surprised them, however (Werner & Smith, 2001). Their situations had improved dramatically. Fewer than 10% had persistent mental health problems or criminal records; the majority (75%) were satisfied with their job performance, social relationships, and marriages; and none was unemployed or on welfare. Most worked in service jobs or as skilled technicians, and half had undertaken further education after high school. By age 40 the same 75% continued to enjoy successful adaptation to the challenges of adulthood. The men were working as skilled workers or technicians in construction, and the women were engaged predominantly in service jobs or health care. Most were very satisfied with their lives.

This outcome is surprising and remarkable, given the very grim start to these children's lives, their predominant social disadvantage, and their troubled and unhappy school careers. To quote Werner and Smith

(2001), "Truly, the 'odds were against them,' yet with few exceptions they have grown into responsible adults who hold down a steady job, have stable marriages and are caring parents" (p. 139). This story is not one of bleak outcomes but of individuals with a desire for a successful life, who apparently understood that they could be more successful in the world of employment and family than they had been in their demoralizing lives as students.

Werner and Smith (2001) identified factors that protected children who overcame their early problems: a temperament that elicited positive responses from caring people around them, special skills and talents, mothers who nurtured self-esteem, supportive adults outside the family who helped them find their path to a satisfying future, and opportunities at major life transitions. Like Morrison and Cosden (1997), Werner and Smith point out "the need to *look beyond the horizons of special education* to ways in which we can provide a continuum of services that reduce the likelihood of negative chain reactions associated with a learning disability" (p. 140, emphasis added). In other words, interventions need to be oriented toward the potential developmental cascade, not just the discrete skill.

The children of Kauai teach another key lesson: Children whose skill set may be ill adapted to the very narrow and specific academic requirements of school can be well adapted as adults for the more diverse world of work, if they can identify their niche. Yet school can be so discouraging, at times irrelevant, and blind to their assets that it can take many years for them to recover a sense of self-efficacy and find their way.

The Frostig Center

These same themes emerged from another study, which collected the life stories of children who had attended a school for the learning disabled. The Frostig Center was established in 1951 in California by Marianne Frostig, well before the learning disability diagnosis was formalized and accepted. Researchers wanted to find out what had become of children who had left the school between 1958 and 1965, when they became young adults, and subsequently as mature adults. In this era preceding the formal acceptance of learning disabilities, these students were likely to have been severely affected. In contrast to the Kauai sample, these children mostly came from families with significant economic resources, who had the means to support the substantial private school tuition.

The children were followed up 10 years (Spekman, Goldberg, & Herman, 1992) and then 20 years after they left the school (Goldberg,

Higgins, Raskind, & Herman, 2003; Raskind, Goldberg, Higgins, & Herman, 1999). Although this project was not as large or methodologically sophisticated as the Kauai study and the children were not representative of the population, its conclusions echoed those of the Kauai study.

At 10 years after graduation, when the children were between 18 and 25 years old, the researchers classified the young adults as either successful or not successful based on a collection of life tasks (e.g., employment, education, family relationships, community relations/interests). They then identified the factors that accounted for success or lack of success. There were surprisingly few differences between the groups in quantifiable background variables, such as cognitive ability, academic achievement, or socioeconomic status. What primarily differentiated them were what the researchers called "success attributes." Specifically, successful young adults had made a realistic adaptation to their learning problems, had greater self-awareness of their problems and how they affected them, were more proactive and persevering, and were more emotionally stable. They were also good at setting goals for themselves and pursuing them. Finally, these people had effective supports (e.g., family members, other supportive adults or peers), and they used these supports well.

Ten years later, that is, 20 years after these individuals had left the school, the researchers once again contacted them, obtained current academic and cognitive testing, and explored further the "success attributes" that they had previously observed (Goldberg et al., 2003). Perhaps the most significant finding from the entire study emerged from the participants' responses to a simple question: "Rate in retrospect how stressful the learning disability was during different periods in your life." The trajectory of this rating tells the essential story: The learning disability was highly stressful in elementary school, then declined in adolescence and even more in adulthood, becoming relatively minor by the time of the interviews (Figure 4.1). Thus, rather than becoming more disabling, as parents so often fear, the reverse was actually the case! The stress of the learning disability in the early years seemed to have cascading effects for many children, involving frequent changes of school, the need to make new friends, and teasing from peers. Even though their academic skills had continued to improve, these adults' skills nonetheless remained quite diminished (only 10th-grade reading level and 9th-grade math). Thus, the stress levels did not decline because they had outgrown the learning disability; rather, these people had discovered niches and strategies for themselves that made academic skills less of an issue. Once school was out of the picture, they found ways to be productive and satisfied with their lives that allowed them to draw on their strengths.

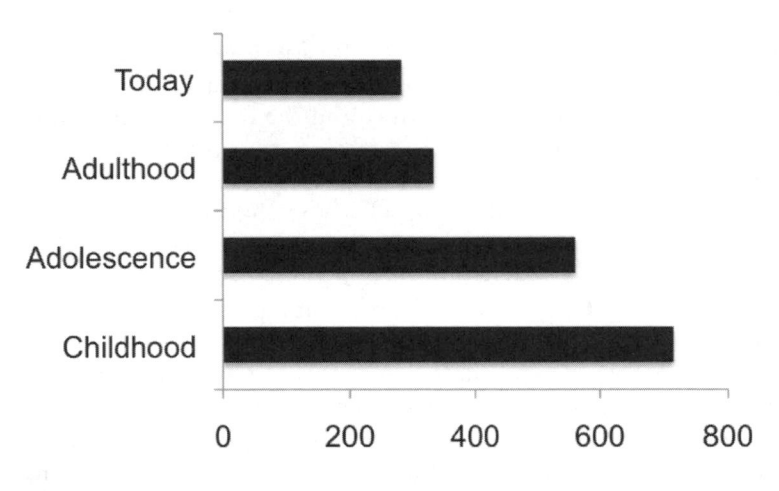

FIGURE 4.1. Retrospective ratings among adults, on a scale of 0 to 1,000, of the stressfulness of a learning disability during different life periods. From Raskind, Goldberg, Higgins, and Herman (1999, Table 2). Copyright 1999 by the Division for Learning Disabilities of the Council for Exceptional Children. Adapted by permission.

In terms of successful adaptation to adulthood, as in the Kauai study, there was considerable continuity over time; individuals who had been unsuccessful at 10 years had not changed their status at 20 years. Despite their academic difficulties, approximately half the individuals had attended college and a quarter had graduated. Whereas 75% were still living with their parents at year 10, this number had dropped to 42% by year 20, a number that is still high relative to the general population. There was a high rate of psychiatric disturbances (approximately 40%), but these diagnoses also did not differentiate the groups. The researchers speculated, however, that special education settings during the era when these people had attended the Frostig School were much more likely to have included children with significant comorbid behavioral or emotional problems.

Again, at 20 years, quantifiable background variables generally did not discriminate the groups. What did discriminate clearly were the same "success attributes"—self-awareness, proactivity, perseverance, goal setting, and use of support systems. These personal attributes were actually far more closely linked to adult success than were IQ, academic achievement, life stressors, age, gender, socioeconomic status, or ethnicity. Noting this primary finding, the researchers comment provocatively, in the vein of Morrison and Cosden (1997), that "one might question the validity of approaches that *focus almost exclusively on remediation of academic deficits*" (p. 46).

COMMENTARY

Several key themes emerge from these studies. First, a learning disability, whatever its specifics, has a *developmental course*. Children are most distressed by their learning disabilities in the early years of school. As time goes on, for many, especially after they leave school, the learning issues are of less concern, as they choose vocations for which their skill set is more appropriate. As these individuals settle into adulthood, they find their niche, and their successful adaptation is related as much to personal qualities as to academic skills. Moreover, early adulthood appears to be a watershed developmental moment in terms of adaptation; in both studies, those who were doing well in their 20s continued to do well, and those who were not doing well did not recover.

Second, and related, children can be protected from risks as they mature into adulthood by the *social context*, primarily supportive adults (parents and other key adults), and *personal qualities* (perseverance, other nonacademic skills, insight into themselves). Although a learning disorder is a risk, other important factors can either diminish or exacerbate its impact. Third, although impaired academic skills are an important piece of the picture, *academic skills are only one component,* and broader personal and ecological factors can have a far more significant impact on life outcomes.

A developmental approach conceptualizes learning problems as an issue of *adaptation*, rather than as a discrete deficit in need of repair. A child's ability to successfully adapt to the demands of schooling depends in part on his or her complement of skills (including academic skills, of course), attitudes, emotions, and proclivities and in part on the demands of the environment. When learning problems are defined in this way, what then does the child with learning problems look like? The next chapter reviews research that addresses this question.

Chapter 5

Identifying Learning Disabilities

A Developmental Approach

But the testing didn't show anything....

Many families bring their children for an independent evaluation because of frustration with school testing. They believe that there is something wrong, and often the teachers agree, but since the test scores do not document a problem, the child cannot be "identified" and thus there can be no tangible response. As a result, families can be left perplexed and frustrated, wondering what categorical and legally recognized box might fit their child so that he or she can get needed help. They go in search of a diagnosis, seeking a solution to their problem. Very often, someone—a teacher or a pediatrician—raises the possibility of "ADD," even though the parent does not feel strongly that attention is the issue. Yet it may be the best available approximation to an appropriate check-box that will allow someone to do something about the problem. If we can understand these children more clearly, we may be able to make better sense of the problem of identification more broadly.

Ironically, the massive body of research on learning disabilities provides remarkably little insight into such children. The same issues that can exclude them from access to special education resources—that is, their apparently "adequate skills" on standard psychoeducational tests—also exclude them from research studies, thereby perpetuating the prevailing systems. Moreover, despite the absence of deficient test scores, it can be apparent that the interaction between the child and the world of school is not going well. These children, whose skills fall in this gray area, often present the greatest challenge in terms of identification and management. This chapter summarizes some of my group's research findings relevant to this group of children. A complete list of publications from this project is provided in the Appendix. The chapter that follows discusses relevant insights from cognitive neuroscience.

A DEVELOPMENTAL APPROACH TO LEARNING DISABILITIES RESEARCH

For our studies, we included children *based solely on the fact that they had been referred for evaluation,* rather than including or excluding children based on achievement test criteria for "specific learning disability." Within this frame of reference, the *referral itself* is the primary behavioral indicator of the dysfunctional interaction, and referral for evaluation thus becomes *the cardinal symptom of disorder.*

From the perspective of research methodology, referred samples are routinely frowned upon, and for good reason. Clinic-referred samples are typically biased, that is, unrepresentative of the population at large. The truth of the matter, though, is that *any* strategy that a researcher applies to include or exclude people from research studies will inevitably entail bias, be it explicit or implicit. Researchers who include only children with poor reading or math skill based on a standardized test will necessarily *exclude* children who have legitimate, cognitive-based difficulties meeting academic expectations but who manage to achieve adequate scores on the particular test. Because the typical research strategies are referenced to skills, the very children who can be most perplexing rarely participate in studies.

The exclusion of such children from studies has undoubtedly contributed to the disconnect cited previously between research-identified children and children who are actually identified by schools and parents as having learning problems. Moreover, for the child and family, the psychosocial impact of school problems may be no different, whether the child meets research criteria or not. Indeed, in some cases the situation may be worse for the child who fails to meet standard criteria because there is no clear and socially acceptable attribution for the struggles and failures. Thus, although our approach necessarily entailed one type of bias, it allowed us to learn more about these children who have received little, if any, systematic attention from researchers, but who are so frequently a source of tension between parents and schools.

In the research program that formed the basis for our studies, we recruited 8- to 11-year-old children who had been referred to a hospital-based program for children with learning problems. Children were evaluated at the point of recruitment and then followed 2 years later. As indicated above, the only criterion for *inclusion* was that the child had been referred for evaluation; actual scores on reading or math tests were irrelevant to eligibility. Because we were interested primarily in idiopathic learning problems (i.e., learning problems that are presumed to be developmental in origin and not due to a medical or psychiatric condition or brain injury), we excluded children who had a history of neurological impairment, who met criteria for ADHD with hyperactivity, who had clinically significant levels of behavioral and emotional problems, or whose IQ was below 80. Children who met criteria for ADHD–inattentive subtype (i.e., without hyperactivity) were retained, since we suspected that these children had underlying cognitive problems that masqueraded as an attention disorder, and we wanted to study them. The non-learning-impaired (NLI) group was composed of schoolchildren from communities with comparable demographic characteristics (e.g., age, sex, parent education, occupation). Children from both groups, not surprisingly given the referral bias, lived primarily in suburban or exurban communities.

The children completed an extensive battery of standard neuropsychological and academic tasks, as well as neurophysiological (EEG and ERP) studies. Reflecting our developmental orientation, a unique feature of the research program was a computer-administered information-processing battery. The tasks measured the integrity of very basic, or "low-level," information processing. Harking back to our discussion of Karmiloff-Smith's framework (1998) in Chapter 3, these "low-level information-processing" (LLIP) tasks may reflect subtle *domain-relevant* biases that evolve developmentally to become manifest behaviorally. These processes, in fact, proved highly relevant to the clinical presentations.

DIAGNOSING THE SKILL VERSUS DIAGNOSING THE INTERACTION

Three studies were focused specifically on children referred for evaluation whose academic achievement, as measured by standard tests, was adequate. That is, they scored in the average range or better, but nonetheless continued to struggle. We called these children *learning impaired–normal achievers* (LI-NA). This LI-NA group comprised approximately *one-third* of our total referred sample, a substantial proportion.

Clinical Neuropsychological Profiles of the LI-NA Group

We first evaluated the performance of the LI-NA children on a standard battery of neuropsychological tests (Morgan, Singer-Harris, Bernstein, & Waber, 2000). In order to do so, we divided the referred sample into two groups:

1. *Learning impaired–low achievers* (LI-LA): Children who scored low (standard score below 90) on at least one screening test of academic achievement (Wechsler Individual Achievement Test [WIAT] Basic Reading, Reading Comprehension, Spelling, or Calculation).
2. *Learning impaired–normal achievers* (LI-NA): Children who scored within normal limits (above 90) on all four WIAT academic tests.

In terms of their demographic characteristics (Table 5.1), the LI-NA group was, as might be expected, more economically advantaged: The parents of these students were better educated and had higher-status occupations. Age at referral was comparable for the LI-NA and LI-LA group, on average in the second to third grade, and approximately 70% of each group was male. Children in the LI-NA group were more likely to attend private school (LI-NA, 38% vs. LI-LA, 10%); less likely to have been evaluated in school, even if they attended public school (LI-NA, 52% vs. LI-LA, 88%); and less likely to be receiving special educa-

TABLE 5.1. Demographic Characteristics of Learning-Impaired–Normally-Achieving and Learning-Impaired–Low Achieving Groups

	LI-NA (n = 40) Mean (*SD*)	LI-LA (n = 81) Mean (*SD*)
Sex	27 M, 13 F	59 M, 22 F
Study age (months)	113.81 (13.9)	116.41 (14.5)
Grade	3.45 (1.2)	3.52 (1.3)
Father's age	42.90 (5.6)	41.91 (5.8)
Father's education (years)*	15.82 (2.7)	14.82 (2.3)
Father's occupation*	7.25 (1.7)	6.45 (1.9)
Mother's age*	41.33 (3.9)	39.72 (4.6)
Mother's education (years)*	16.00 (2.2)	14.63 (2.1)
Mother's occupation*	7.27 (1.6)	6.55 (1.6)

Note. Sex reported as frequencies, not means. Two-tailed t-test for group difference. LI-NA, learning impaired–normally achieving; LI-LA, learning impaired–low achieving. Data from Morgan et al. (2000).
*p < .05.

tion services (LI-NA, 45% vs. LI-LA, 74%). The private school statistics in part reflect greater economic means among the LI-NA children's families. In our experience, however, many families do not enroll their children in private or parochial school primarily because they believe in private education. Rather, they may recognize the child's academic vulnerability, have the means for school tuition, and hope that smaller classes or more rigorous structure will protect the child from "falling through the cracks."

Eighty percent of the LI-NA group was referred for learning problems, but only 43% for a reading problem (10% spelling, 38% math). Thus, although they were having learning problems, parents tended not to focus on a specific skill deficit as the source of the problem. In contrast, for the LI-LA group, 98% were said to have a learning problem, and reading was among the primary complaints for 87% of them (65% spelling, 26% math).

On first blush, it appears that the adequate achievers may simply be children whose overly concerned families have the resources to seek an evaluation or finance private schooling, but who did not have a *real* problem. Their neuropsychological test performance, however, suggested otherwise. As Figure 5.1 shows, in terms of basic measures of IQ and academic achievement, the *profiles* of the LI-NA and LI-LA groups are remarkably similar. Although the LI-NA group has higher scores across the board, their strengths and weaknesses track in parallel.

Next, we examined the performance of the LI-NA group on other clinical neuropsychological measures. Although their IQ (mean = 111) was above the expected mean of 100 for the population, the LI-NA group performed only at the average level on measures of visuomotor integration and verbal memory, and more poorly on verbal fluency, graphomotor output, rapid automatized naming, and copying a complex design (Rey–Osterrieth Complex Figure). In fact, the *only* functions that were *above* the population mean, like their IQ, were single-word reading, nonword reading, and reading comprehension (all untimed). Apparently, their *primary* area of relative competency, in addition to general cognitive ability, was untimed reading. Reading efficiency was less competent, but still in the average range. For the LI-NA group, competent reading skills may have masked underlying difficulties. In a world where reading is accorded a privileged position as a benchmark for identification and access to special education resources, these children could easily elude detection.

Perhaps, though, these adequate achievers simply represented a brighter and more socially advantaged group for whom the classic discrepancy definition of learning disability (i.e., between IQ and achievement) would identify the problem. Although 35% of the LI-NA group

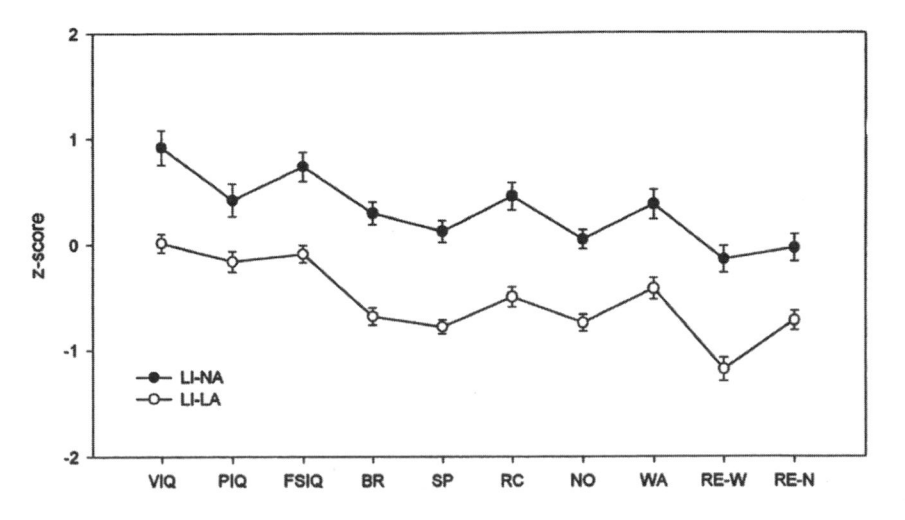

FIGURE 5.1. Mean scores for IQ and academic achievement measures expressed as z-scores by group. LI-NA, learning impaired–normal achieving; LI-LA, learning impaired–low achieving; VIQ, WISC-III Verbal IQ Scale; PIQ, WISC-III Performance IQ Scale; FSIQ, WISC-III Full Scale IQ; BR, WIAT Basic Reading; SP, WIAT Spelling; NO, WIAT Numeric Operations; WA, Woodcock–Johnson Word Attack; RE-W, reading efficiency—words; RE-N, reading efficiency—nonwords.

actually did meet criteria for an IQ–achievement discrepancy (on any achievement measure), this discrepant subgroup performed no differently than the rest of the LI-NA group on the neuropsychological measures. Children without the discrepancy exhibited just as much difficulty processing information as did those who demonstrated the discrepancy. Thus, the IQ–achievement discrepancy is not especially useful as an identification strategy, as has long been argued (Fletcher et al., 1994), even in this brighter than average group.

Next, we compared the LI-NA and LI-LA groups to each other on the neuropsychological measures. In order to do so, we first adjusted all the neuropsychological test scores statistically for the effect of IQ. By so doing, we equalized the groups for general cognitive level. Figure 5.2, which shows the results, highlights two findings. First, the profiles are again remarkably similar, the main differences emerging on measures that are most sensitive to linguistic and symbolic competence. Second, once the scores have been adjusted for IQ, the performance of the LI-NA group is consistently below par; that is, they are performing more poorly than expected based on their IQ. As an aside, one cannot help but be

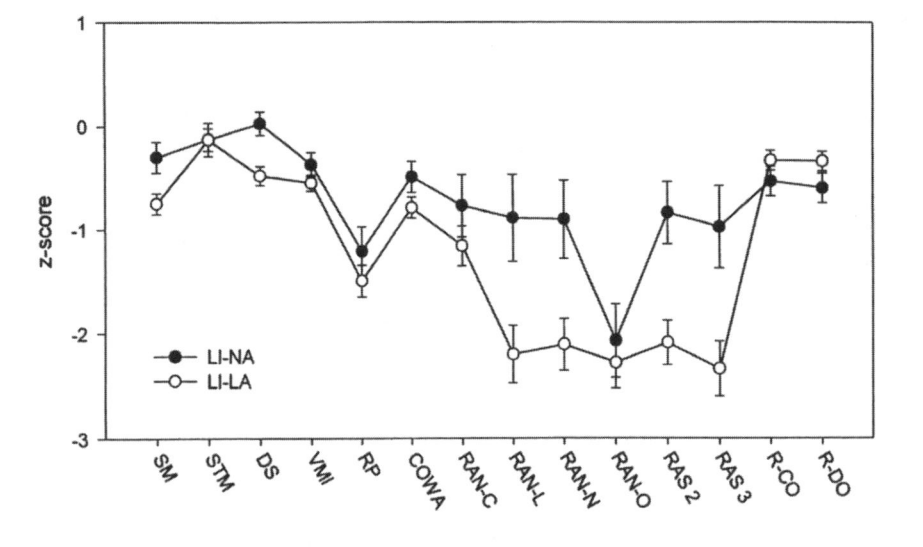

FIGURE 5.2. Mean scores adjusted for Full Scale IQ for neuropsychological measures expressed as z-scores. LI-NA, learning impaired–normal achieving; LI-LA, learning impaired–low achieving; SM, WRAML Sentence Memory; StM, WRAML Story Memory; DS, WISC-III Digit Span; RP, repeated patterns; COWA, controlled oral word association; RAN-C, rapid automatized naming colors; RAN-L, rapid automatized naming letters; RAN-N, rapid automatized naming numbers; RAN-O, rapid automatized naming objects; RAS-2, rapid alternating stimuli 2-set; RAS-3, rapid alternating stimuli 3-set; R-CO, Rey–Osterrieth Complex Figure Copy Organization; R-DO, Rey–Osterrieth Complex Figure Delayed Recall Organization.

struck by the fact that both groups show a diverse array of problems that certainly extend well beyond discrete academic skills.

The largest differences between the LI-NA and LI-LA groups emerged for rapid automatized naming (RAN) (Denckla & Rudel, 1976). On this task, the child is asked to read 5 stimuli (letters, numbers, colors, or pictures) arrayed randomly and repetitively in 5 rows of 10 items. The score is based on the number of seconds taken to complete the reading of each stimulus card. The LI-LA group performed extremely poorly on these tasks, clearly worse than the LI-NA. Even so, when compared to population norms, the scores of the LI-NA group were still *one to two standard deviations* below average for age, even without adjusting for IQ. Their fundamental information processing was thus legitimately compromised, even though they performed adequately on standard tests of discrete academic skills, especially if efficiency was not considered. In general, their problems were most pronounced on tasks sensitive to *effi-*

ciency of information processing and *managing complexity and information load.* These fundamental cognitive capacities can be invisible to standardized tests of discrete academic skills, yet can interfere with a child's ability to manage more complex day-to-day demands of the curriculum. They may well bring the child to clinical attention, especially in schools where the curriculum is more fast-paced and demanding, because of the dysfunction in the interaction between the child and the world of school.

Thus, both groups have valid reasons to be struggling in school, especially relative to their social context, and their cognitive profiles are surprisingly similar. The LI-LA group is performing more poorly in general, especially on language-related tasks. They also come from somewhat lower socioeconomic backgrounds, with potential impact on language development. In this study, however, lower socioeconomic status was relative and did not necessarily connote economic disadvantage. Parents of the LI-LA children had, on average, nearly 3 years post high school education, compared to an average of 4 years for parents of children in the LI-NA group, not dramatically different. Once we venture beyond the safe harbor of reading or math scores, it is difficult indeed to decide (1) who does or does not have legitimate claim to a learning disability or even (2) what a learning disability is.

Low-Level Information Processing in Referred Adequate Achievers

As alluded to above, a key innovation of our studies was a computer-based test battery that measured LLIP. Theoretically, these tasks provide a window into the integrity of the basic building blocks of information processing. Because they are all novel to the child and nonverbal, they should be relatively independent of language experience and instruction. They are also extremely simple, with performance measured by button-press responses, timed to milliseconds, on tasks that are administered via computer.

As suggested above, performance patterns on these tasks may reflect subtle biases, domain-*relevant* features of neurobehavioral development (Karmiloff-Smith, 1998). Of course, as Gottlieb (Gottlieb & Halpern, 2002) cautioned, genetic and experiential processes in behavioral development are essentially inseparable. We should not assume, therefore, that these low-level processes are a mapping of genetically determined risk. The LLIP measures can, however, be reasonably understood as neurodevelopmental markers of risk for learning problems.

Figures 5.3 to 5.6 briefly describe the four tasks. (Detailed descriptions can be found in the original published reports.) Because the tasks

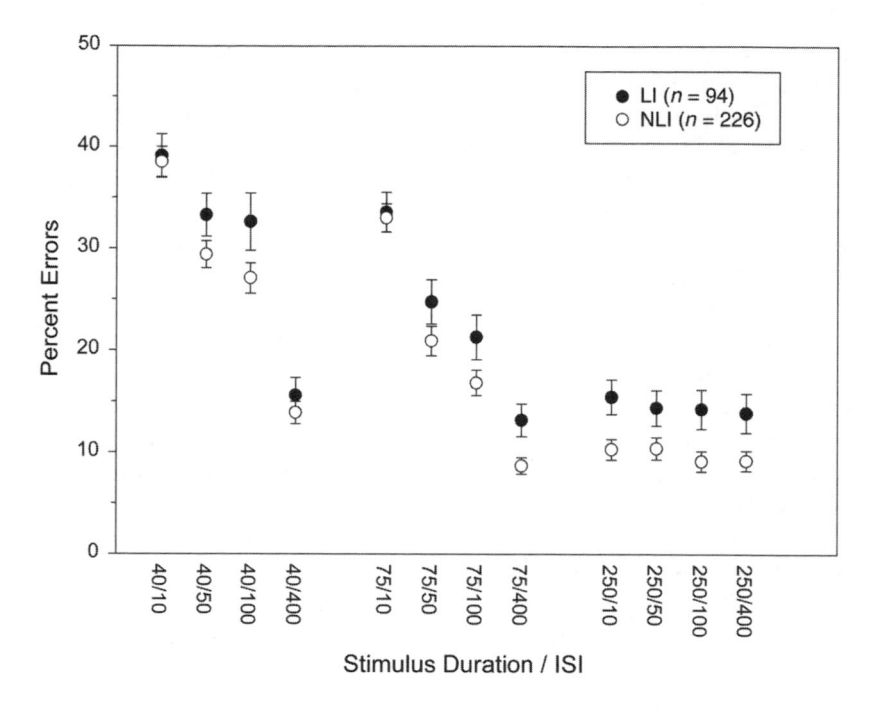

FIGURE 5.3. Rapid auditory processing. This task was modeled after the task described by Tallal (1980). Children were presented with brief complex tones (one low and one high). The tones were presented in pairs (e.g., low–low, low–high), and the children were asked to signal by button press whether the tones were same or different. Stimulus length ranged from 40 milliseconds to 250 milliseconds, and the interstimulus intervals (ISIs) ranged from 10 milliseconds to 400 milliseconds. The outcome was *number correct*. The figure illustrates mean total errors for learning-impaired (LI) and non-learning-impaired (NLI) children by stimulus duration and ISI. Children in the learning-impaired group generally made more errors; a higher error score indicates poorer performance.

are inherently repetitive and tedious, requiring many presentations of similar stimuli, we borrowed a page from video game developers, embedding these boring tasks in a fantasy video game format (a space adventure or an underwater adventure). The fantasy element proved highly engaging and kept the children motivated to persist for the roughly 10 minutes required for each task.

The clinical neuropsychological testing had indicated that the cognitive profiles of the LI-NA and LI-LA groups were similar, although those of the LI-NA group were less severe. Standard clinical neuropsychological tests involve relatively complex functions. Exam-

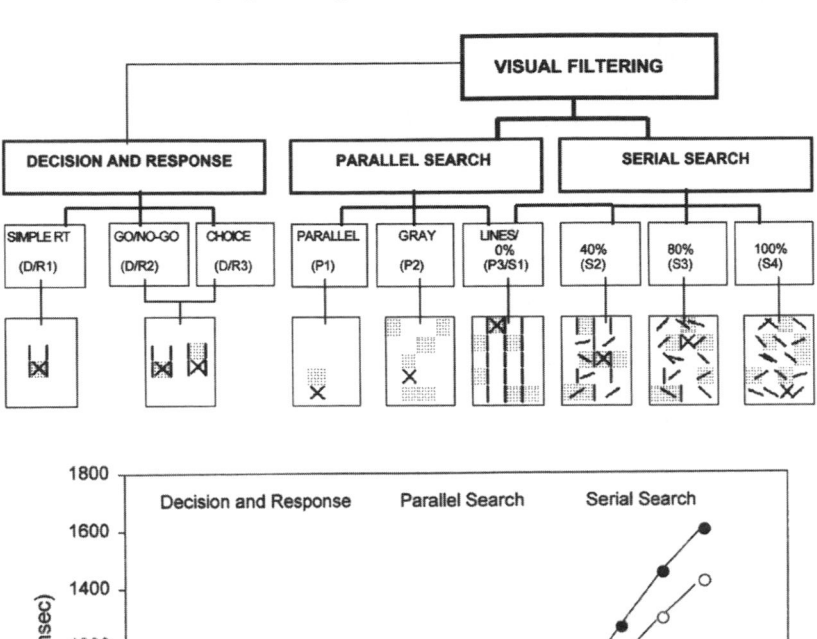

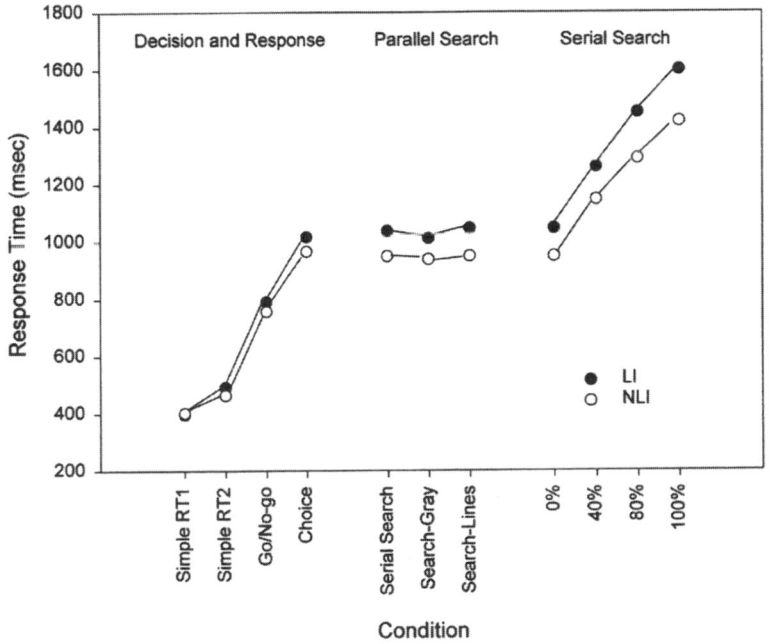

FIGURE 5.4. Visual filtering. This task measures speed of visual serial search (Weiler, Harris, et al., 2000). It requires that the child determine whether an "X" is located on or off a gray shape. Line fragments are superimposed, and their location and orientation are varied from 0% fragments random (parallel) to 100% fragments random (most visual clutter). As the proportion of randomly oriented line fragments increases, the time to sort through the visual clutter and accurately report whether the "X" is on or off the gray shape increases. The outcome was *response time*. Learning-impaired children showed longer response times, especially as the visual clutter increased.

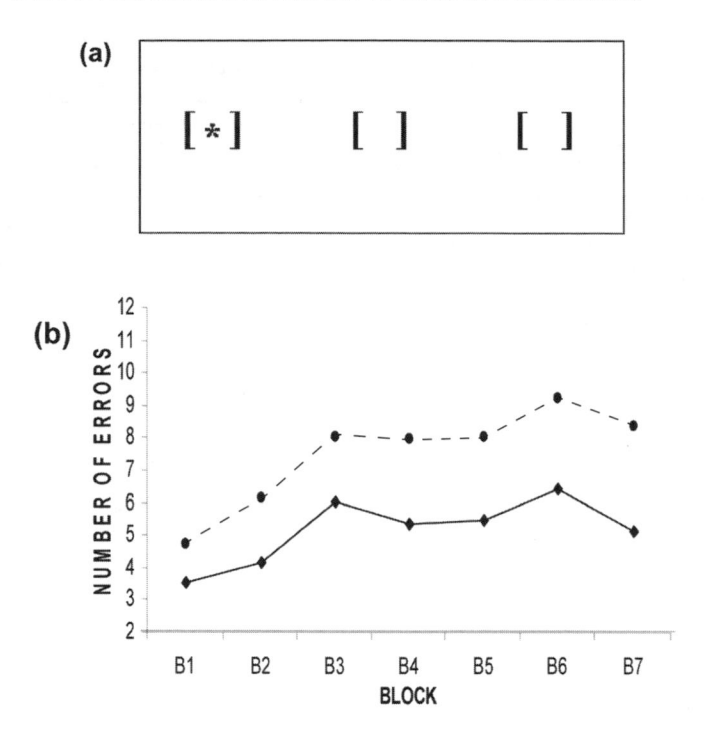

FIGURE 5.5. Motor sequence learning. This task measures implicit learning of motor sequences (Nissen & Bullemer, 1987). Children press keys corresponding to the changing location of a stimulus in a visual display, depicted in the Figure 5.5a. The location of the stimulus changes in a repeating sequential pattern; with repetition, response times typically improve, indicating that learning has occurred, even though the child may have no conscious knowledge of a sequence. Learning is "implicit." After a number of sequenced trial blocks, a block in which the stimuli are presented in random order is presented. If the child's response times become longer, it is inferred that the prior decrease in times reflected implicit learning of the motor sequence. The outcome was measured in terms of *number of errors*. Both good and poor readers showed increased errors on the random block (B6), but poor readers made more errors overall in Figure 10.5b (from Waber, Marcus, et al., 2003).

ining the performance of these children on the LLIP battery, however, allowed us to measure the integrity of information processing at a more basic level, glimpsed on a scale of *milliseconds* rather than minutes or even seconds.

For this study (Singer-Harris, Forbes, Weiler, Bellinger, & Waber, 2001), we compared the LI-NA children with peers from the community, who were matched not just for age, sex, and IQ but also for their *single-*

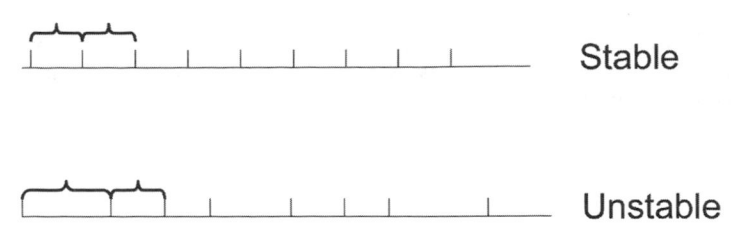

Stable

Unstable

FIGURE 5.6. Paced finger tapping. This task was modeled after the finger-tapping task of Wolff (Wolff, Michel, Ovrut, & Drake, 1990). Children learn to finger-tap bimanually, that is, alternating their hands, in time to the beat of a metronome, and are instructed to continue tapping after the metronome is turned off. The outcome of interest is the stability of the rhythm, as measured by *variability of the intertap intervals* when the child taps without the metronome. The figure above illustrates a stable and unstable tapping pattern; unstable patterns yield higher scores. Children with learning impairment showed less stable tapping patterns (Waber, Weiler, et al., 2000).

word reading scores. Word recognition is generally regarded as the most fundamental and reliable indicator of reading impairment. With reading accuracy, a primary signifier of learning disability, held constant, would these information-processing tasks still differentiate the referred LI-NA children from their nonreferred peers? We included children from the LI-LA group in this study as well, matched to the LI-NA group for age, sex, and nonverbal cognitive ability, allowing us to inquire whether the information processing of the adequate achievers was more like that of the reading-matched community controls or the low-achieving children, whose reading was poorer. Characteristics of these groups are shown in Table 5.2.

Figure 5.7 shows the three groups' performances on the information-processing tasks. (Note: A *higher* score indicates *poorer* performance.) For all four tasks, the scores of the LI-NA group fell midway between the community control group and the LI-LA group. Statistically, the LI-NA group performed more poorly on the battery as a whole (average score for the four LLIP tasks, or LLIPAVG) than did the reading-level-matched community controls ($p < .05$), but their scores *did not differ statistically* from those of the LI-LA group ($p = .51$). Here again, now at the level of very *basic information processing*, the LI-NA group performs more poorly than the matched controls, even though the students in this group read as well as their peers, and their general cognitive ability is comparable!

School-Referred Children?: A Community-Based Study

We next examined the meaning of referral for evaluation focusing just on the community group, a more epidemiological strategy that is less

TABLE 5.2. Demographic Characteristics and Intelligence and Achievement Scores by Group and for the Total NLI Sample for Low-Level Information-Processing Comparison

	LI-NA (n = 65)	LI-LA (n = 65)	NLI (n = 65)	All NLI children (n = 243)
Sex	41 M, 24 F	43 M, 22 F	36 M, 29 F	107 M, 136 F
Age	9.6 (1.7)	9.5 (1.2)	9.5 (1.1)	9.4 (1.2)
Parent ed*	31.4 (4.7)	29.4 (3.6)	30.5 (4.5)	29.7 (4.6)
Parent occ*	14.1 (3.2)	12.9 (3.3)	13.1 (3.5)	12.8 (3.6)
K-BIT				
V*	107.4 (11.1)	99.1 (10.1)	109.3 (9.0)	109.2 (10.4)
M	106.0 (12.8)	104.3 (12.2)	107.2 (9.4)	109.4 (14.4)
C*	107.4 (10.6)	102.0 (9.2)	109.2 (8.4)	110.4 (11.6)
WIAT				
BR*	104.9 (9.8)	88.8 (9.4)	105.8 (8.6)	108.6 (11.8)
SP*†	102.8 (9.2)	87.6 (7.9)	106.4 (8.2)	108.9 (10.6)
NO*†	101.2 (7.6)	88.5 (10.7)	107.8 (8.8)	108.2 (11.5)

Notes. Except for sex, means are reported with standard deviations in parentheses. LI-NA, learning impaired–normal achieving; LI-LA, learning impaired–low achieving; NLI, non-learning impaired; Parent ed, parent education, total number of years for parents combined; Parent occ, parent occupation, total Hollingshead (1975) rating for parents combined; K-BIT, Kaufman Brief Intelligence Test (V, Vocabulary; M, Matrices; C, Composite); WIAT, Wechsler Individual Achievement Test (BR, Basic Reading; SP, Spelling; NO, Numerical Operations). Data from Singer-Harris et al. (2001).

*LI-NA versus LI-LA $p < .05$, two-tailed t-test.

†LI-NA versus NLI $p < .05$, two-tailed t-test.

vulnerable to the criticism of referral bias (Waber, Marcus, et al., 2003). Two years after their initial recruitment and evaluation, we ascertained which children had been referred for school evaluation during the interim. We could then review our data retrospectively to see how the referred children had performed on our test protocol *prior to* their referral. These "community-referred" children were compared to three other groups: (1) peers from their community who had not been referred (community nonreferred); (2) peers from their community who had already been identified as needing special education at the time of the initial recruitment to the study (community special education); and (3) children in the clinic sample (clinic referred).

Of the 178 children from the community, 17 (11%) had been referred for school evaluation during the 2 intervening years, 14 of whom were subsequently provided some form of special education. Table 5.3 shows the characteristics of each group at study entry. Several points are noteworthy. First, the mean scores of the community-referred children are virtually identical to the population mean of 100 for both cognitive abil-

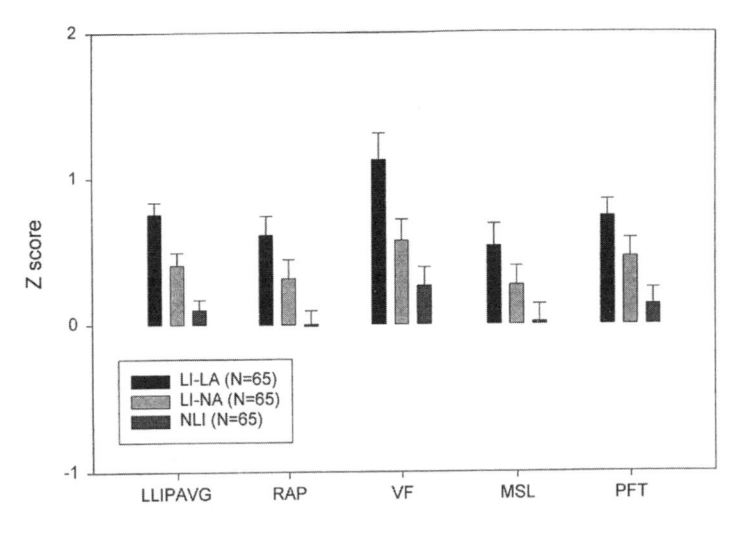

FIGURE 5.7. Means and standard errors of scores by group on LLIP tasks. LI-LA, learning impaired–low achieving; LI-NA, learning impaired–normally achieving; NLI, nonlearning impaired; LLIP, low-level information processing; LLIPAVG, average LLIP score across four tasks; RAP, rapid auditory processing; VF, visual filtering; MSL, motor sequence learning; MTC, motor timing control. From Singer-Harris, N. et al. (2001). Children with adequate academic achievement scores referred for evaluation of school difficulties: Information processing deficiencies. *Developmental Neuropsychology, 20*(3), 593–603. Copyright by Taylor & Francis Group. Reprinted by permission.

ity and achievement, and they are also entirely comparable to those of children in their community who had already been identified for special education. This finding corroborates the contextual nature of the special education identification process (Bocian et al., 1999). Allocation of special education services can be a function of relative need as much as of objectively referenced test scores. The scores of the nonreferred peer group from this community, however, are *above* average by the same objective criteria. Thus, performance that is exactly average by some formal norm-referenced criterion may be functionally deficient *in that community*. Only the clinic-referred group has mean achievement scores that are significantly below expectation by the more objective performance criteria. This pattern reinforces the notion that the clinically identified "problem" does not reside in some decontextualized and objectively specifiable disability that is contained within the child, but arises from a problem with the *interaction* between the child and the environment, which is further influenced by locally referenced considerations of relative need.

TABLE 5.3. Means and Standard Deviations (in parentheses) for Cognitive Ability, Achievement, Low-Level Information Processing, and Attention Measures for Community-Referred, Community-Non-Referred, Community Special Education, and Clinic-Referred Groups at Time 1

Measure	CNR (n = 161)	CR (n = 17)	CSE (n = 30)	CLR (n = 145)
K-BIT Verbal	111.1 (9.2)[a]	100.8 (9.6)[b]	101.3 (10.0)[b]	102.8 (11.1)[b]
K-BIT Matrices	110.5 (13.7)[a]	97.7 (11.8)[b]	101.8 (13.7)[b]	102.9 (12.8)[b]
K-BIT Composite	**112.1 (10.6)**[a]	**99.2 (10.2)**[b]	**101.8 (11.4)**[b]	**103.2 (10.5)**[b]
WIAT Basic Reading	109.9 (11.1)[a]	101.7 (13.9)[ab]	97.9 (14.2)[b]	94.9 (12.8)[b]
WIAT Spelling	109.9 (10.5)[a]	102.2 (8.3)[b]	96.8 (13.6)[bc]	92.5 (11.5)[c]
WIAT Numerical Operations	108.4 (10.7)[a]	100.2 (10.4)[ab]	97.5 (14.6)[b]	91.6 (11.5)[b]
Achievement	**109.4 (8.8)**[a]	**101.4 (6.8)**[b]	**97.4 (12.1)**[bc]	**93.0 (9.9)**[c]
Motor Timing Control	−0.1 (1.0)[a]	0.5 (1.1)[ab]	0.4 (1.0)[ab]	0.6 (0.9)[b]
Rapid Auditory Processing	0.0 (1.0)[a]	0.7 (1.3)[ab]	0.4 (1.2)[ab]	0.7 (1.2)[b]
Motor Sequence Learning	−.1 (0.8)[a]	0.9 (0.9)[b]	0.5 (1.5)[b]	0.4 (1.3)[b]
Visual Filtering	−0.1 (0.9)[a]	0.70 (1.0)[b]	0.80 (1.0)[b]	0.90 (1.3)[b]
Information Processing	**−0.1 (0.6)**[a]	**0.7 (0.8)**[b]	**0.5 (0.9)**[b]	**0.6 (0.7)**[b]
Parent—Inattention Scale	4.8 (4.0)[a]	10.6 (7.2)[bc]	9.4 (5.9)[b]	12.7 (5.9)[c]
Teacher—Inattention Scale	3.8 (4.2)[a]	10.0 (6.0)[b]	12.2 (8.3)[b]	12.1 (7.1)[b]
Inattention	**4.3 (3.4)**[a]	**10.3 (6.1)**[b]	**11.2 (6.6)**[b]	**12.4 (5.7)**[b]
Parent—Hyperactivity Scale	3.8 (3.6)[a]	7.8 (6.6)[b]	4.5 (3.7)[a]	6.6 (5.0)[b]
Teacher—Hyperactivity Scale	3.5 (4.5)[a]	5.9 (5.9)[a]	3.6 (4.4)[a]	5.6 (5.5)[a]

Note. Variables in **bold** are primary summary outcome scores. **Achievement,** mean of WIAT scores; **Information Processing,** mean of low-level information-processing scores; **Inattention,** mean of Parent and Teacher DRS Inattention scales; CNR, community nonreferred; CR, community referred; CSE, community special education; CLR, clinic referred; K-BIT, Kaufman Brief Intelligence Test; WIAT, Wechsler Individual Achievement Test; Hyperactivity and Inattention Scales are raw sum of ratings for scale items. Overall group effects significant at $p < .001$ level for all variables with the exception of teacher hyperactivity ($p < .05$). From Waber, D. P., et al. (2003). Neurobehavioral factors associated with referral for learning problems in a community sample: Evidence for an adaptational model for learning disorders. *Journal of Learning Disabilities, 36*(5), 467–483. Copyright by Sage Publications, Inc. Reprinted by permission.

[a,b,c]Means with different superscript letters are significantly different ($p < .05$) after Bonferroni adjustment for multiple comparisons and adjustment for age and sex.

Table 5.3 also shows the LLIP (information processing) scores of the four groups. The mean scores of all three referred groups are elevated (i.e., poorer) relative to the norm for the community. Similarly, the behavioral ratings for inattention are elevated in all three clinical groups. Perhaps these children have as yet unidentified ADHD. Yet only 1 of the 17 community-referred children met DSM-IV clinical criteria for ADHD–inattentive subtype and none for the hyperactive or combined subtypes. It is unlikely, therefore, that the children in this group "just" had undiagnosed ADHD. Behaviors that would lead an observer to endorse symptoms of inattention could easily reflect inefficient information processing (e.g., avoids mental effort, makes careless mistakes). Significantly, for both laboratory measured information processing and ecological behavior ratings, this community-referred group cannot be distinguished from the community special education or clinic-referred groups.

So why were these children referred? Perhaps these were "just average" children living in an "above-average" world. Alternatively, if the referral reflected sensitivity to some compromise of basic information processing, the referred children should also differ in terms of their attention behaviors and information processing from nonreferred peers from the same schools performing *at the same academic levels*. To examine this question, we matched the 17 community-referred children with 17 nonreferred peers for age, sex, and overall academic achievement (average of all the WIAT achievement scores).

Table 5.4 shows the results of this comparison. In fact, factors other than basic academic skills did distinguish these children. The nonreferred children had higher cognitive ability scores, perhaps helping them to compensate for their average skills. Ironically, the nonreferred children actually demonstrated a *larger* discrepancy between ability and achievement than did the referred children! Yet the same nonreferred children also displayed significantly better information processing (almost exactly at the mean for their community), shown on the right side of the table. Moreover, they exhibited fewer inattention symptoms, not appreciably different from the rest of the nonreferred sample who had, on average, much better academic skills. Apparently, if we regard the referral as a marker of dysfunction in the child–world interaction, these information-processing characteristics and their manifestations in day-to-day functioning carry considerable weight in raising questions about the child's ability to navigate the academic setting, over and above basic academic skill levels as measured by standardized psychoeducational tests. So it was not just a matter of lower academic achievement

TABLE 5.4. Means, Standard Deviations (in parentheses) and *t*-Tests for Matching Variables and Outcome Variables for Community-Referred and Community-Non-Referred Groups

	Community-referred group	Community-non-referred group	t	p
Age (months)	9.1 (1.1)	9.2 (0.9)	–.4	.7
Sex (% male)	29.4	35.3	–	1.00#
Achievement	101.4 (6.8)	101.3 (6.7)	–.04	.97
K-BIT Composite	99.2 (10.2)	108.0 (11.2)	2.40	.02
Information Processing	0.7 (0.8)	0.1 (0.4)	–2.64	.01
Inattention	10.3 (6.1)	5.6 (3.6)	–2.70	.01

Note. n = 17. Achievement, mean of WIAT scores; Information Processing, mean of low-level information processing scores; Inattention, mean of Parent and Teacher DRS Inattention scales; K-BIT, Kaufman Brief Intelligence Test. From Waber, D. P., et al. (2003). Neurobehavioral factors associated with referral for learning problems in a community sample: Evidence for an adaptational model for learning disorders. *Journal of Learning Disabilities, 36*(5), 467–483. Copyright by Sage Publications, Inc. Reprinted by permission.
#Fisher's exact test.

scores relative to the local norm, but lower academic achievement scores *in combination with* less efficient basic information processing, and, potentially, compensatory reasoning skills. These studies illustrate both the contextual nature of learning disability identification, as well as the domain-general aspect of the problem—that is, having a more generalized impact on functioning than just discrete reading or math skills.

SOME CONCLUSIONS

Our research confirmed that many children who are referred for evaluation but obtain scores on achievement tests that are adequate by standard psychoeducational testing can nonetheless possess legitimate neurocognitive barriers to adaptation to curricular demands, especially when referenced to their particular social and educational context. For our clinic-referred adequate achievers, IQ was above the population mean, yet performance on most neuropsychological measures lagged behind IQ and was well below even the population mean for a number of measures. Moreover, their neuropsychological profile was remarkably similar to that of the low-achieving group, although their scores were at a higher level, in general. Information-processing efficiency and integration of more complex information stood out as primary impediments to school success for these children.

Several conclusions can be drawn from these studies. First, the data reinforce the notion that the problem rests in the interaction between the child and the environment and is not *contained* within the child; the phenomena are contextually dependent. Children referred for evaluation who were not "low achievers" by formal test criteria tended to come from more advantaged backgrounds, in the context of which their performance appeared more discrepant because the demands may have been greater. However, the problem was not simply one of being an average child in an above-average world. When we matched referred children to nonreferred children from the community with the same achievement levels, the referred children were further distinguished by less efficient information processing as well as behaviors that are generally viewed as symptoms of inattention. These "inattentive" behaviors could plausibly reflect inefficient processing. Indeed, the children in our study who *did* meet DSM-IV criteria for the inattentive subtype of ADHD were distinguished not by difficulty sustaining attention over the course of a long and tedious task, but by slow information processing (Weiler, Bernstein, Bellinger, & Waber, 2002).

The distinction between adequate-achieving and low-achieving referred children appears to be one of *degree and context rather than difference*, the notable exception being untimed reading. Standardized achievement tests, which typically measure discrete learned skills, can often fail to capture the problems with which these children contend. These problems tend to involve fluency, efficiency, output, and (for want of a better word) integration, and are remarkably similar in both adequate and low achievers. These associated problems can interfere with the child's ability to implement his or her skills and to meet academic demands, especially online in a classroom.

A comprehensive appreciation of the child, not as a collection of skill packets but as an individual developing systemically within a context, can often help to modify dysfunctional interactions. Doing so within a legal and administrative structure that assumes discrete skill deficits can be difficult, however. Too often, everyone seeks a simple diagnostic label that is expected to somehow provide prescriptive answers (e.g., a particular reading program, a medication). Within a more developmental model, whether children do or do not "have" a learning disability becomes less relevant; the question is whether the child's complement of skills and dispositions is such that he or she can reasonably adapt to the socially determined demands that that particular child encounters, and then how to adjust the "child–world" system to make the adaptation more successful.

Finally, our research found inefficient information processing to be a surprisingly unifying feature among many children who are referred for evaluation, whether or not specific skill deficits can be documented by standardized testing. The next chapter considers what this finding may mean in light of insights derived from contemporary cognitive neuroscience.

Chapter 6

Insights from Cognitive Neuroscience

Automatic and Effortful Processing

It's like he just needs to work harder for everything
he gets....

The research described in the previous chapter leads to the bold claim that the single cognitive feature that best distinguishes children with learning impairment from their peers is not their reading, math, or writing skills, per se, but their inefficient information processing. The referred children were variable in their performance on screening tests of academic achievement, with some in the average range and some below it. Their most unifying feature, however, was inefficient information processing, as measured by a computerized assessment battery. Along these lines, in our study of rapid automatized naming (Waber, Wolff, Forbes, & Weiler, 2000), roughly 70% of children referred for evaluation of their learning exhibited abnormally slow naming speed for letters and numbers, regardless of their particular learning problem (e.g., reading, math, attention). No matter how we approached the question, the result was always the same: *Children referred for evaluation, whether or not they had identifiable academic skill deficits by standardized achievement testing, were far more likely than peers to exhibit inefficient information processing.*

Contemporary cognitive neuroscience provides insight into potential sources of this inefficient processing, highly relevant for our dilemma. In this chapter we review key studies and relate them to findings from our own research. The research reviewed below by no means provides clear answers, but it does suggest theoretical frameworks and mechanisms that can reorient our thinking about these children in novel ways. These frameworks, moreover, link nicely to the developmental science discussed at length in Chapter 3.

COGNITIVE EFFICIENCY: CONTROLLED AND AUTOMATIC INFORMATION PROCESSING

In a classic series of papers, Schneider and Shiffrin elaborated a theory of automatic and controlled information processing (Schneider & Shiffrin, 1977; Shiffrin & Schneider, 1977). These papers were to have a profound influence on cognitive psychology over the next several decades. Hasher and Zacks (1979) referred to these constructs as *automatic* and *effortful* processing, labels that nicely fit the phenomena we observe in children with learning problems. These processes are fundamental to human performance, in general, and to the cognitive functions of central concern in children with learning disorders in particular. According to Hasher and Zacks, "Operations that drain minimal energy from limited-capacity attentional mechanisms are called *automatic*. Automatic operations function at a constant level under all circumstances, occur without intention, and do not benefit from practice." In contrast, "*effortful* operations, such as attentional capacity, interfere with other cognitive activities also requiring capacity, are initiated intentionally, and show benefits from practice" (p. 356).

Cognitive neuroscientists seeking to understand brain mechanisms underlying these core phenomena are now extending that work using functional neuroimaging tools. To quote one group of investigators (Jansma, Ramsey, Slagter, & Kahn, 2001):

> Because controlled processing calls upon a capacity limited system, the shift from controlled to automatic processing is essential in order to free up resources needed for more complex tasks (Carlson, Sullivan, & Schneider, 1989; Schneider & Fisk, 1982a, 1982b). The ability to automate task processing may therefore be essential for complex task execution, as it enables reallocation of limited attentional and processing resources. (p. 730)

When we undertake a new task or learn a new skill, at first we rely almost exclusively on effortful processing, deploying conscious resources to plan and organize our efforts and make our way through whatever it is we are trying to learn. With experience or practice, however, we shift all or part of the function to more automatic processing. Learning tennis or keyboarding are familiar examples of such a shift, but automaticity figures in more complex cognitive functions as well, such as learning to use a new computer program or play chess, or more to the point here, learning to read text or perform multistep calculation. Automatic processing is thus essential for cognitive development and performance. *From the perspective of understanding children with learning problems, the significance of this automatic–effortful distinction cannot be over-emphasized.* The neuroscientific studies described below focus on the automatic–effortful dimension in the context of two cognitive functions that are well known to be affected in children with learning disorders: working memory and processing speed.

HOW DOES THE BRAIN SHIFT
FROM CONTROLLED TO AUTOMATIC PROCESSING?

The shift from controlled to automatic processing has been repeatedly demonstrated behaviorally, but what actually happens in the brain during this shift? Jansma and colleagues (2001) set out to address just this question. Building on a well-researched working memory paradigm in cognitive psychology, known as the Sternberg task (Sternberg, 1966), they sought to identify neural correlates of the shift from controlled to automatic processing. Specifically, they used fMRI to compare activation patterns associated with the same task under novel and practiced conditions. In the version of the task adapted for fMRI (Figure 6.1), the participant sees a display of 5 letters, which is then taken away, followed by a series of 10 letters presented one by one. The person presses a button to indicate whether each of the single letters was or was not included among the 5 in the display. In the *novel* condition, which requires controlled processing, a new set of 5 letters is presented before each run of 10 test trials; in the *practiced* condition, which facilitates automatic processing, the same 5-letter set is displayed before each set of test trials.

Behaviorally, in the practiced condition (compared with the novel condition), response latencies and variability decreased while accuracy increased—hallmarks of the shift to automatic processing. The primary question is, what occurred in the brain? The experiment identified seven regions that were activated by the novel task, involving prominently left dorsolateral prefrontal cortex, supplementary motor area, and parietal cortex, regions typically activated by working memory paradigms. The key finding, however, was that *in the more automatic, practiced condition, the extent of activation was reduced in all seven regions.* No particular region or regions were associated with the shift, nor was the

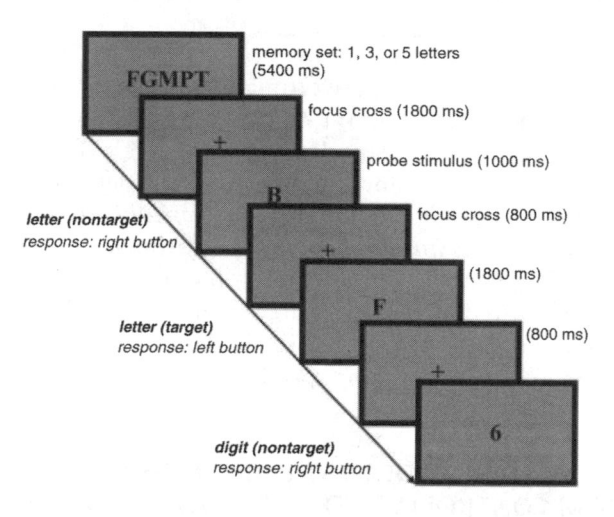

FIGURE 6.1. Schema for fMRI working memory task. From Jansma, J. M., et al. (2001). Functional anatomical correlates of controlled and automatic processing. *Journal of Cognitive Neuroscience, 13*(6), 730–743. Copyright by the Massachusetts Institute of Technology. Reprinted by permission.

functional network restructured, which would have signaled shifting of the automatized function to other regions. Rather, with benefit of practice, the entire network appeared to function more efficiently, leading to "reduced claim on the capacity-limited WM system" (Jansma et al., 2001, p. 736).

The adaptive significance of this increased efficiency is apparent. To again quote the authors (Jansma et al., 2001) "Cognitive functioning is generally based on a complex balance between automated and controlled processes" (p. 739). To the extent that functions require controlled processing, and thus access to capacity-limited resources, those resources will not be available for other cognitive functions, potentially undermining higher-order cognitive processes. Such a system may be less capable of meeting more complex challenges, especially those entailing greater information load, and of integrating component operations in the service of higher-order functions. This study thus provides a glimpse of what kind of brain mechanisms might underlie variations in automatization, as well as sensitivity to complexity or information load, that we see clinically in so many children with learning problems.

HOW DOES AUTOMATIZATION RELATE TO COGNITIVE CAPACITY AND PERFORMANCE?

A subsequent study examined whether the ability to automatize, as manifest physiologically on fMRI, would correlate with more effective behavioral utilization of limited processing capacity (Ramsey, Jansma, Jager, Van Raalten, & Kahn, 2004). Processing capacity is classically measured by dual-task paradigms (e.g., walking and chewing gum at the same time!). The logic is as follows: A person is asked to perform a task, and the performance is measured. The individual repeats the task, but this time simultaneously with another task that competes for processing resources. The decrement in performance in the primary task is regarded as an index of processing capacity.

In this particular study, adult volunteers performed the working memory task described above in the MRI scanner, in both the novel and practiced conditions, and the extent of practice-induced reduction of neurophysiological activity was quantified. They then performed another working memory task, this time involving tones, in the scanner. The activation maps documented overlap between the visual and auditory working memory tasks in several key regions (left dorsolateral prefrontal cortex and anterior cingulate cortex), establishing a framework of competition for resources.

After the scanning session, participants were asked to perform the visual and auditory tasks again, this time simultaneously. As expected, in this dual-task condition, they made more errors, indicating that they had exceeded capacity limitation. Most significantly, however, *individuals who demonstrated greater signal reduction in the brain scans as a result of practice with the task made fewer errors on the primary task* ($-.78, p = .003$). Thus, the ability to shift to more efficient and automatic neural processing, measured neurophysiologically, was manifest functionally as more effective use of limited capacity. The authors suggested that the practice effect reflects a "trimming" of neuronal ensembles. Practice, they suggest, may have induced a *disengagement of neurons whose action is not relevant for mapping the correct responses onto the given stimulus*, resulting in a more streamlined and efficient system.

This scenario should sound familiar. In Chapter 3 we reviewed the interactive specialization model (Johnson, 2001), in which a similar process is posited to occur developmentally. In the course of the child's experiential interaction with the environment, pathways that have intrinsic structural advantage are more consistently activated by a particular functional demand, whereas less well-suited pathways become committed to other functions for which they are better adapted. As these pathways are repeatedly used for particular functions, they become entrenched and committed, resulting in the more modular and efficient functional organization of the adult brain. Recall our friends Joe and Don becoming increasingly specialized as their company grew and accordingly integrating their separate functions in service of the goals of the company. The specialization and integration dynamic described in Chapter 3, now being demonstrated developmentally in the neuroimaging research, is fundamental to the ability to manage more complex and challenging information. Equally important, it resonates with the clinical presentation of many children with learning problems, who need to invest deliberate effort to accomplish tasks that peers may accomplish with minimal focused attention and effort.

Similarly, at the "micro" level of task performance, this neurophysiological trimming apparently can occur during new learning throughout the lifespan. Just as specialization of function facilitates integration of multiple component processes, the ability to automatize and streamline networks may facilitate switching between multiple contexts (in the case of dual-task interference) and, more importantly, can free up limited cognitive resources in order to accomplish more complex cognitive goals. Significantly, practice-related decreases in the extent of activation are linked to improved communication between elements of the network, which is in turn associated with more efficient learning (Buchel, Coull, & Friston, 1999). It would not be unreasonable to expect that the ability to trim or streamline these networks in the learning process is related to the ability to do so developmentally, as networks are being constructed. Moreover, these characteristics may not be limited to one functional domain but appear to be more broadly distributed. This framework could have significant bearing on our understanding of the ontogeny of learning disorders and, in particular, the pervasive problems with efficiency and integration.

NEURAL SUBSTRATES OF PROCESSING SPEED

The above discussion raises the core issue of communication among component elements of networks, which presumably enhances efficiency. Clinically, children with learning disorders, including ADHD, typically show slower processing speed than peers (Ho & Decker, 1988; Tiu, Thompson, & Lewis, 2003; Weiler, Wolff, et al., 2000; Willcutt, Pennington, Olson, Chhabildas, & Hulslander, 2005). Information-processing efficiency, moreover, is fundamental to both cognitive development and higher-order cognitive performance (Kail, Weinert, & Schneider, 1995; Verhaeghen & Salthouse, 1997). The neural mechanisms underlying processing speed, and especially individual variation in this capacity, are thus germane to the problem of learning disorders.

The Coding subtest from the Wechsler scales has been most consistently and reliably used to measure processing speed in children. In this task the child is presented with a page, at the top of which is a code table, consisting of the digits 1–9 arrayed in a row of boxes, with a nonsense symbol in the box below each digit. The rest of the page displays rows of randomly sequenced digits, each with an empty box beneath it. The child has 2 minutes to correctly fill in as many empty boxes as possible in sequence.

Although the clinical significance of this task has long been recognized, its neurobiological underpinnings have been poorly understood. Rypma and colleagues (2006) adapted the task for fMRI, providing insight into the basis for individual and perhaps even developmental variation in performance on this key task. In the paradigm developed for the scanner, the code table was shown at the top of each display, with a single digit–symbol pairing displayed below it (Figure 6.2). The participant pressed a button indicating whether the probe pairing did or did not match one of the pairs in the code table. Response time in the scanner correlated well with performance outside the scanner on the standard Digit Symbol test, the adult version of the Coding subtest, confirming that the scanner version was a good proxy for the clinical test.

As is standard in fMRI studies, areas of increased activation were identified. Of greater interest for the present discussion, however, were

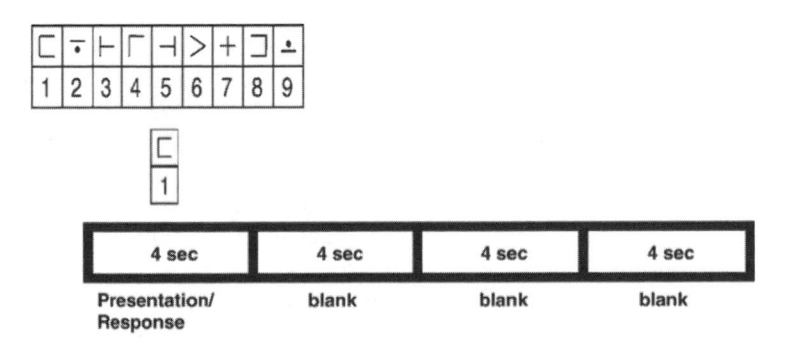

FIGURE 6.2. Trial-sequence of the modified Digit Symbol (Coding) paradigm for fMRI study. On each trial a novel code table appeared in the middle of the screen while a probe digit–symbol pair appeared below it. Stimuli remained on the screen for 4 seconds followed by variable intertrial intervals (0, 4, 8, or 12 s). From Rypma, B., et al. (2006). Neural correlates of cognitive efficiency. *NeuroImage, 33*(3), 969–979. Copyright by Elsevier. Reprinted by permission.

causality analyses that quantified to what extent activation data recorded from a region in the functional network at one point in time predicted data recorded from another region at a later point in time. These analyses provide insight into the functional network, especially the streamlining process associated with automatization or fluency in the execution of the task.

The fMRI analysis identified areas of activation in the left dorsolateral prefrontal cortex (DLPFC) and bilateral parietal cortex. As Figure 6.3 shows, these two regions were differentially related to performance speed. Whereas greater extent of DLPFC activation was tightly linked to *longer* response times ($r = .88$, $p < .001$), the opposite was true for the parietal regions ($r = -.76$, $p < .004$). Greater extent of activation in parietal cortex was associated with *shorter* response times.

The causality analyses clarified the meaning of this finding. The investigators hypothesized that for slower performing individuals, prefrontal (executive) systems guide posterior (integrative) systems, but that the reverse is true of faster performers. To test the hypothesis, they contrasted causality analyses for the four individuals with scores above the median for the group on the Digit Symbol test and the six individuals with the scores below the median.

Figure 6.4 illustrates three striking findings. *First*, the individuals with slower processing speed exhibited many more interregional influences than the faster ones, consistent with better streamlining of the network among participants who achieved higher scores. *Second*, as hypothesized, slower individuals showed more causal relationships directed from frontal to parietal cortex than did the faster individuals. Indeed, more projections from the DLPFC to the other regions predicted longer response times ($r = .60$, $p < .003$). *Third*, the slower individuals also showed more reciprocal connections between the DLPFC and other regions ($p < .01$), again complicating and presumably compromising the efficiency of the system (Figure 6.5).

This study provides insight into sources of processing inefficiency, especially meaningful because the task paradigm has direct clinical significance for developmental learning disorders. Indeed, in our own study of referred children described in Chapter 5 (Morgan, Singer-Harris, Bernstein & Waber, 2000), Wechsler Intelligence Scale for Children–III (WISC-III) Processing Speed index scores were consistently lower than scores on Verbal Comprehension and Perceptual Organization, whether children were adequate or low achievers.

The Rypma study suggested that "efficient interregional communication provides the neural basis of processing speed" (Rypma et al., 2006, p. 976). Efficient interregional communication was also associated with decreased extent of activation in the DLPFC. In contrast with the work-

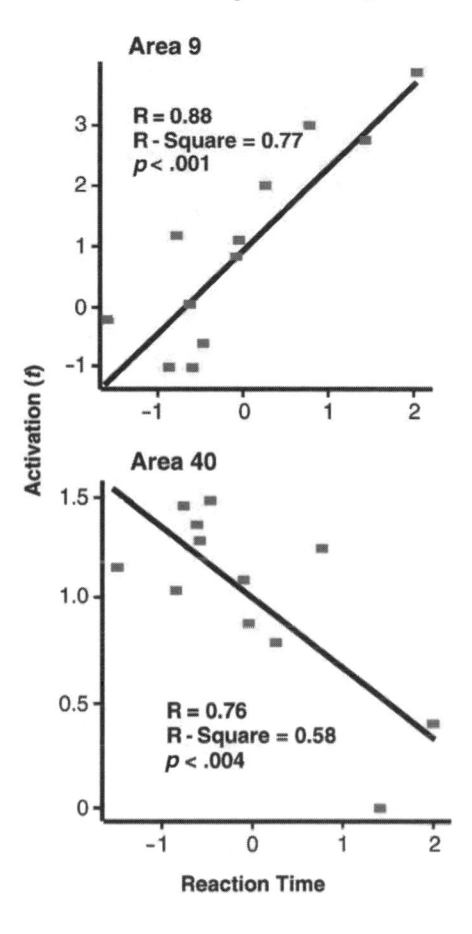

FIGURE 6.3. Results of regression analyses between region-of-interestwise cortical activity and reaction time (RT). Scatterplots show regional mean *t* values for each individual plotted against their standardized RTs. Activation increases in area 9 (prefrontal cortex) with longer RTs; activation decreases in area 40 (parietal cortex) with longer RTs. From Rypma, B., et al. (2006). Neural correlates of cognitive efficiency. *NeuroImage, 33*(3), 969–979. Copyright by Elsevier. Reprinted by permission.

ing memory studies outlined above, however, here greater efficiency was also associated with *more* activation in the parietal cortex. In discussing their findings, the authors suggest that more fluent performance occurs when the parietal cortex and the ventromedial prefrontal cortex can support visual search with minimal executive control. Slower performance occurs when greater DLPFC involvement is required to guide other brain

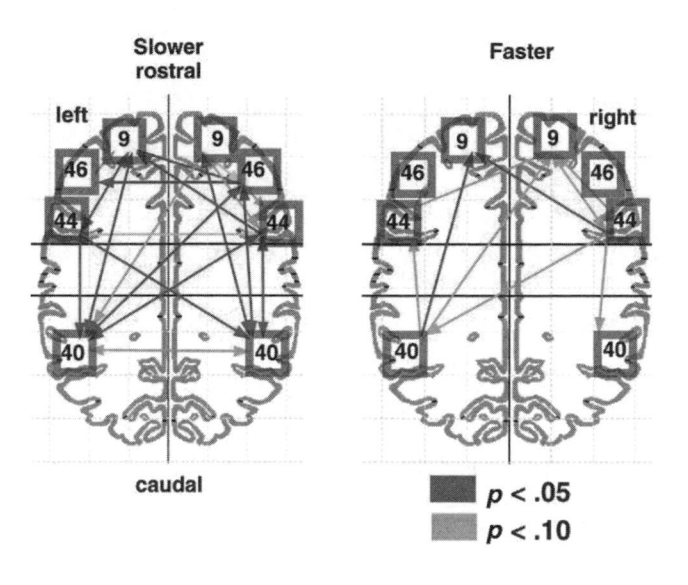

FIGURE 6.4. Results of causality analyses between prefrontal (Brodmann areas 9, 46, and 44) and parietal (Brodmann area 40) regions. Influences were calculated separately for faster and slower individuals (grouped by median split; arrows indicate significant influences; dark arrows = $p < .05$; lighter arrows = $p < .10$). From Rypma, B., et al. (2006). Neural correlates of cognitive efficiency. *NeuroImage, 33*(3), 969–979. Copyright by Elsevier. Reprinted by permission.

regions (controlled or effortful processing). More broadly, the quality of the interaction between parietal and frontal regions may be another neural mechanism underlying variation in automatization or efficiency and thus may have important implications for learning disorders.

The most telling outcome, however, is the causality analysis, vividly illustrated by the figure: the network underlying fast performance is clearly more streamlined and efficient. The quality of functional (and perhaps structural) connectivity between brain regions, most likely related to a process of interactive specialization in development, should thus be high on our list of potential mechanisms underlying the decreased efficiency that is so common among children with learning problems and may offer clues to their heterogeneous functional problems.

The studies described to this point indicated that a shift to more automatic processing often entails reduction in brain activity, which can literally free up capacity for other purposes. This reduction of activity, moreover, likely signals trimming or streamlining of the functional neural network. To bring this line of reasoning full circle, we return to the children described in Chapter 5.

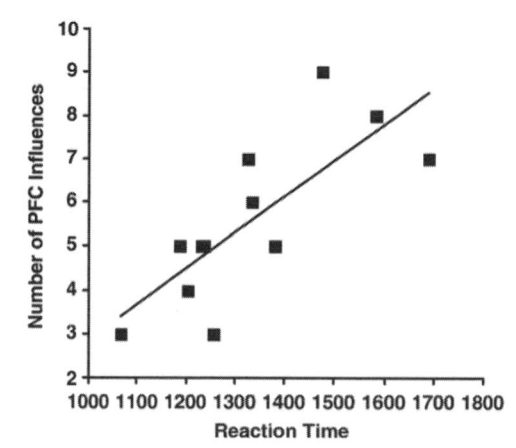

FIGURE 6.5. Scatterplot of connectivity–performance relationships. Number of Brodmann area 9 (prefrontal) influences (those extending from Brodmann area 9 to other regions identified by the causality analysis) plotted against individual subjects' RTs (slope = .77; r_2 = .60; p < .003). From Rypma, B., et al. (2006). Neural correlates of cognitive efficiency. *NeuroImage, 33*(3), 969–979. Copyright by Elsevier. Reprinted by permission.

CONNECTIVITY IN CHILDREN REFERRED FOR EVALUATION OF LEARNING PROBLEMS

Our research program included a neurophysiological ERP study designed to address the issue of connectivity (Peters, Waber, McAnulty, & Duffy, 2003). ERPs were recorded while children performed a simple nonverbal information-processing task. Arrow stimuli of three types were presented: left-pointing, right-pointing, or a horizontal line with straight lines instead of arrows on its ends (Figure 6.6). If the arrow pointed to the left, the child was to press the left key on a button box; if it pointed to the right, the child was to press the right key; and if there were no arrows, the child was to refrain from doing anything. Correct and incorrect responses, response times, and brain activity were all recorded.

The study mapped the time course of processing in relevant brain regions, to which EEG is exquisitely sensitive. In particular, the goal was to evaluate *temporal coupling* of activity in these regions as the task was being performed in order to examine whether referred and nonreferred children might display differential connectivity patterns at this very fundamental level of information processing. A technique called event-related correlation (ERC) was used to detect this temporal coupling. Similar to the causality analyses described above, time-lagged cor-

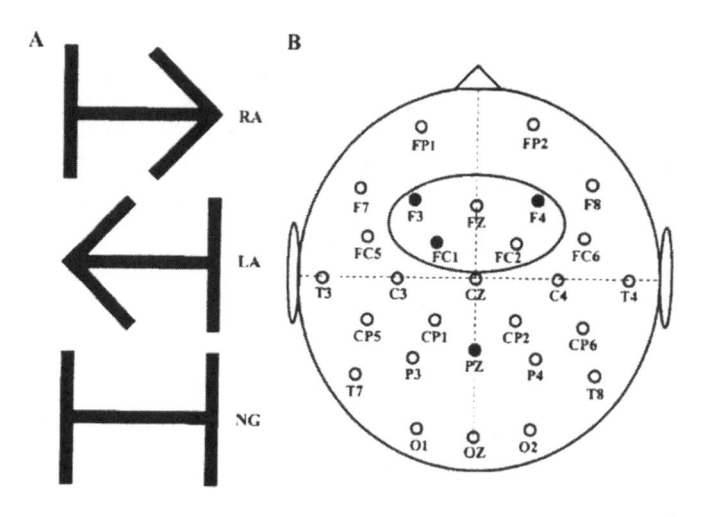

FIGURE 6.6. (A) Three visual stimuli for paradigm. When the stimulus labeled RA (right arrow) appeared, the child pressed a button in the right hand. When the LA (left arrow) stimulus appeared, the child similarly pressed the left button. When the NG (no-go) stimulus appeared, no response was to be made. (B) Schematic head in vertex view with left ear to the left and nose above. Event-related correlation (ERC) was formed and analyzed between PZ and all electrodes within the inner oval region encompassing electrodes F3, FZ, F4, FC1, and FC2. From Peters, J. M., et al. (2003). Event-related correlations in learning impaired children during a hybrid go/no-go choice reaction visual–motor task. *Clinical Electroencephalography, 34,* 99–109. Copyright by the EEG and Clinical Neuroscience Society. Reprinted by permission.

relations were performed between regions, with waveforms recorded at one time point correlated with waveforms recorded at later time points from other relevant brain regions. The magnitude of these correlations would index temporal coupling between regions.

Motor action is controlled primarily in the left frontal region of the cerebral cortex, whereas visual input is processed bilaterally in the posterior regions. Figure 6.6 shows the placement of electrodes on the head. Activity from the central posterior PZ electrode was correlated in the time-lagged fashion, described above, with activity from the frontal electrodes demarcated by the circle. The filled black circles are regions of interest—that is, regions that are selected on an a priori basis for analysis.

At the behavioral level the groups differed only marginally in their overall accuracy. Also, children responded faster and more accurately to right-pointing arrows (right hand–left hemisphere response) than to left-pointing arrows (left hand–right hemisphere response), consistent with known left-hemisphere control of motor action. The laterality effect was more pronounced among nonreferred children, however, largely because the referred children made more omission errors with their right hand.

The first step in the neurophysiological analysis was to map the temporal course of brain activity associated with the task. At the earliest stage of processing (30–50 milliseconds), the right arrow elicited coupling of the left anterior motor region (F3) with PZ, while the left arrow elicited coupling of the PZ region with the right anterior motor region responsible for the left hand response (F4). These associations presumably reflected enhanced input of visual information to the relevant motor area. Somewhat later in time, but prior to the motor response (50–60 milliseconds), another association emerged, coupling PZ with FC1, also in the left frontal regions, this time for both the right- and left-pointing stimuli. This later activity may have reflected the go/no-go decision.

Of greater interest, however, were the correlations between these ERCs, which signify coupling between regions, and performance accuracy for the referred and nonreferred children. Several important patterns emerged (Table 6.1). First, the PZ–F3 (left hemisphere) feature is correlated with task accuracy for both the left and right arrows. Significantly, however, for the *right-arrow* (*left-hemisphere*) condition, the correlation was present only for the referred group. It emerged for both groups, however, for the left arrow (the correlation was of the same magnitude

TABLE 6.1. Correlation between Behavioral Variables and Region-of-Interest Features for F3 and F4

	Baseline NP-corrected PZ–F3 feature		Baseline NP-corrected PZ–F4 feature	
	Right arrow (RA)	Left arrow (LA)	Right arrow (RA)	Left arrow (LA)
All ($n = 240$)				
Correct	−0.19**	−0.21***	−0.12	−0.14*
Omission	0.18**	0.22***	−0.12	0.15*
LI ($n = 169$)				
Correct	−0.21**	−0.21**	−0.15	−0.14
Omission	0.22**	0.23**	0.22**	0.16*
NLI ($n = 71$)				
Correct	−0.03	−0.22	0.05	−0.11
Omission	−0.02	0.20	−0.06	0.11

Note. From Peters, J. M., et al. (2003). Event-related correlations in learning impaired children during a hybrid go/no-go choice reaction visual–motor task. *Clinical Electroencephalography, 34,* 99–109. Copyright by the EEG and Clinical Neuroscience Society.
*$p < .05$; **$p < .01$; ***$p < .001$.

for both groups but not statistically significant for the nonreferred group because there were fewer subjects). Few significant correlations were detected for the PZ–F4 feature (right hemisphere), most likely because the left hemisphere plays the dominant role in motor planning.

What might these findings mean, especially in light of the fMRI studies? During repetitive tasks, EEG activity decreases over time with practice (Busk & Galbraith, 1975; Gevins et al., 1990), paralleling the decreased extent of activation with practice seen in fMRI studies. As we noted, "The difference [in the correlation patterns] might reflect differential ability to automatize, that is, to routinize simple responses, thereby freeing cortex for other tasks" (p. 108). The referred children may have been less effective at automatizing this exceedingly simple task, resulting in persistent and more extensive cortical involvement, most prominent over the left hemisphere and for the right-hand condition, where the connection should be most direct and thus automatic. Perhaps these findings reflect differences in the ability to streamline the functional network for this very simple task. With the fMRI studies as background, this study suggests why the referred children in our studies so consistently exhibited diminished efficiency for the very simple, nonlinguistic low-level information-processing tasks included in the computer battery.

THE AUTOMATIZATION HYPOTHESIS
IN A DEVELOPMENTAL CONTEXT

This automatization hypothesis is certainly not novel. In 1982 Sternberg and Wagner described "automatization failure" in learning disabilities, referencing the same information-processing framework that is the basis of this discussion. Shortly thereafter, Denckla and Rudel (1976) introduced the Rapid Automatized Naming test, which they viewed as a marker of dyslexia, and the task became a mainstay of dyslexia research. Wolf and Bowers (1999) extended this work in their "double deficit" theory of dyslexia, with decreased automaticity seen as a basis for deficits in reading fluency. Other investigators (Nicolson & Fawcett, 1990; Yap & van der Leij, 1994) implemented dual-task paradigms involving nonreading tasks to advance a hypothesis that an automatization deficit is an integral component of dyslexia (van der Leij & Van Daal, 1999). Nicolson, Fawcett, and Dean (2001) invoked these findings as evidence for a cerebellar hypothesis of dyslexia. More recently, however, Moores, Nicolson, and Fawcett (2003) also situated their hypothesis within this automatic–effortful framework.

As argued in the prior chapter, the growing practice of equating learning disability with a specific skill deficit, giving only minimal attention to other aspects of the child's functioning, can risk fallacious conclusions. An automatization hypothesis of dyslexia may be one of these, despite its considerable contributions to the discussion. Although individuals with reading impairment may, as a group, be less effective at automatization, it turns out that children with learning difficulties are, *in general*, less effective at automatization, whether they can read adequately or not (Waber, Wolff, et al., 2000). Moreover, as detailed in the previous chapter, these information-processing characteristics can distinguish referred from nonreferred children when measures of skill do not. Problems with automatization surely contribute to reading difficulties, but many learning-impaired children have automatization deficits even though their fundamental reading skills are not the most prominent problem.

Since inefficient information processing is so pervasive among children referred for learning problems, understanding its sources is highly relevant. The neuroscientific studies summarized here suggest that automatization is not so much a *skill* as a *process* that pertains to functional networks in general and is integrally related to experience. This process is relevant at both the "macro" developmental level and at the "micro" level of learning.

Within the broader framework of a child–world model, these inefficiencies become functionally problematic to the extent that they are inadequate to meet socially determined goals or to support the acquisition of higher-order skills. As the academic stakes are raised on a social and political basis and as expectations for an independent ability to master more complex and abstract information grow, more and more children will be vulnerable to falling short for reasons that are likely to be highly variable. A century ago, in a society centered on agriculture and manufacturing, such demands were not of particular concern; in a modern information-rich society, however, such inefficiencies can have profound functional significance.

With all of this as background, the assertion that an automatization deficit—or indeed any discrete and focal deficit—"causes" dyslexia or any other learning disorder in some linear cause-and-effect progression should be viewed with caution. Rather, following from Gottlieb's concept of probabilistic epigenesis, the causal mechanisms and outcomes will inevitably be heterogeneous. Were this not the case, we would long ago have reached consensus about the learning disability diagnosis. Instead, the phenomenology of these disorders is largely one of dynamic heterogeneity, determined as much by ecological demands as by a deficit or disability within a child. It is exceedingly unlikely, therefore, that there exists some yet-to-be-discovered biological "silver bullet" that will easily solve the enigma of learning disorders.

CLINICAL IMPLICATIONS

From a clinical perspective, the concepts of automatic and effortful processing are central to the phenomenology of learning disabilities. Although children with learning problems typically display variable and heterogeneous profiles in their specifics, one cannot help but be impressed, when watching them work, by the effort and intention that so many need to invest to execute tasks that peers perform fluently and often effortlessly. The affected tasks typically extend well beyond the declared area of deficit (e.g., reading, math) that brought them to clinical attention. Whether the job is coming up with answers to questions, writing their name, or reciting the months of the year, it often just looks harder. A child may need to invest so much effort in performing academic-type tasks that he or she retains limited wherewithal to interact socially, giving the impression of aloofness or withdrawal. Or a child may become cognitively flooded with information load and respond with anxiety, withdrawal, or restlessness.

Although it would certainly be premature to draw conclusions about specific brain mechanisms based on the little that is known, cognitive neuroscience offers what are best viewed at this point as models or metaphors to guide our appreciation of these clinically relevant phenomena. Concepts such as effortful and automatic processing and streamlining of functional networks, and especially interactive specialization, will shape our understanding of these children in a very different way than the prevalent model of a globally intact child with a discrete modular problem in reading or calculation. The distributed network image, so vividly depicted by the data from the Rypma and colleagues (2006) study, is a powerful one that intuitively rings true as we observe many of these children in action. One child operates with a relatively streamlined complement of efficient interactions, the other with multiple and sometimes conflicting or redundant sources and directions of influence, likely requiring heightened involvement of a central executive—hence "effort." Why this should be the case and how to modify it are key questions for future research. Understanding the etiology of these inefficient networks, however, will surely involve developmental science.

PART II

DIAGNOSING THE CHILD–WORLD INTERACTION

Chapter 7

Identical Twins

> The primary goal ... of the assessment process is not
> to diagnose deficits in a child, but rather to construct a
> Child–World System that characterizes the reciprocal
> relationship of the developing child and the world in
> which that child functions.
> —BERNSTEIN AND WABER (1990)

The cases that follow in Part II of this book illustrate a strategy for translating into practice the developmental approach outlined in Part I. These cases draw on clinical material from the Learning Disabilities Program at the Children's Hospital Boston as well as from the related research program described in Chapter 5. The Learning Disabilities Program is a clinical and training program that employs a developmental neuropsychological approach to analyze the functioning of children with school problems. The children described in this chapter as well as in Chapters 8 and 9 were evaluated in the program. The goal of evaluation, in theoretical terms, is to *diagnose the dysfunction in the child–world interaction* and to provide *strategies for improving it*.

Although the basic developmental principles can be seen in all the cases, each chapter emphasizes different ones. This chapter presents Alexander and Benjamin, identical twins whose stories illustrate how brothers who share 100% of their genetic material and are raised in the same home, can still differ behaviorally, including in their cognitive profiles. Environmental influences lead to both similarities and differences. Their story illustrates concretely the potential for interaction between genetic and experiential processes. Chapter 8 describes Andrew, who exemplifies the "adequate achiever referred for evaluation" group described in Chapter 5. His story illustrates that the dysfunction in the child–world system can elude standard psychometric testing while the unacknowledged dysfunction impacts the child and his family. It also suggests strategies that could facilitate the child–world system without significant investment of resources. Chapter 9 presents Sarah, whose story illustrates how an initial complaint of a "reading problem" can actually signal more systemic compromise, which, if neglected or mismanaged, can cascade and adversely affect academic and social development in far more consequential ways than just reading. It also illustrates how intervention to restore equilibrium to the child–world system can reverse the cascade, with positive effects for the child and family, and likely for the school as well.

Chapter 10 presents the longer-term stories of three children, now young adults, who were evaluated clinically and who also participated in the research program described in Chapter 5. Their stories provide important perspectives on the longer-term developmental evolution and adaptive processes that take place in children with learning problems, as was discussed in Chapter 4. Moreover, they affirm the considerable relevance of risk and protective factors in shaping developmental cascades and, equally important, of a lifespan perspective.

AN OVERVIEW OF THE EVALUATION PROCESS

The Learning Disabilities Program brings together an interdisciplinary team of evaluators with expertise in neurology, neuropsychology, speech–language pathology (oral language), reading and writing (written language), mathematics, and clinical psychology. Children are evaluated in the course of a long morning, rotating among all the specialists. In the afternoon, the team holds case conferences, during which specialists present their findings to one another. Using a hypothesis-testing process, they build a *model of the child–world system.* One team member functions as the case coordinator, leading the team meeting, writing the summary report, and meeting with parents and sometimes school personnel to discuss the findings. Developmental neuropsychological theory informs interpretation of all data, comprehensive of cognitive functioning, academics, and social skills. The integrated formulation then directs development of the intervention plan.

Consistent with the systemic "whole child" focus, every child, no matter what the presenting complaint, completes all components of the evaluation. This is an important element of the process. A child may present with a question of ADHD, but in a systemic model the apparent attention problems may, for example, actually reflect slow processing speed (neuropsychology), impaired language comprehension (speech–language pathology), or anxiety (psychology). A child may present with a concern about reading problems, but the cognitive profile may predict math problems at a higher grade or within the particular curriculum that the school uses. A seemingly pathological presentation on the psychological evaluation may, in fact, reflect the cognitive profile; for example, a child who has difficulty managing complex information can often fail to accurately interpret social cues, leading to social and emotional fallout. Problems with the pragmatic aspects of communication can affect social skills development, potentially compounding school-related anxiety because of aversive peer interactions, or compromising the child's ability to appreciate intention in more advanced texts, and thus affecting reading comprehension. A child's shifting demeanor or consistencies across disciplines can also be revealing. The child who is sullen in the more challenging academic evaluations may brighten in the psychology interview, indicating that an apparently depressed mood is actually situational. Demonstrating areas of strength is as important as demonstrating deficiencies, since strengths are key to constructing the formulation and especially to long-term adaptation.

Since the screening assessments are relatively brief within this format, test protocols are designed to be efficient, and individual evaluations complement one another, with minimal overlap. Tests are essential tools, but they are augmented by careful observation of *how* the child achieves scores as well as the child's spontaneous behavior, demeanor, and interaction style. For the academic assessments, ecologically relevant materials provide insight into how the child manages curricular challenges, over and above discrete skills, which may be intact and thus yield unremarkable scores on standard psychoeducational tests. As evaluators gain experience with these brief protocols, individual variations among children stand out. The evaluator's internal database of performance is established by testing many children using the same relatively brief battery, against which individual differences and patterns of association can emerge prominently. An unusual or unexpected response to a standard question or instruction can often be telling diagnostically. Equally important, as each evaluator builds familiarity with the protocols from other disciplines in case discussions, evaluators can use material from other disciplines to refine their diagnostic hypotheses.

Figure 7.1 shows schematically the components of the evaluation and how they interrelate. A hypothesis about the source of the child's problems is formulated based on the history and tested and modified progressively against findings from each of the disciplines. Elements are confirmed, rejected, or added as the case conference progresses. Hypotheses are tested within a developmental framework; evaluators try to understand how a situation at one point in development could give rise to another later effect within the child's particular context and especially

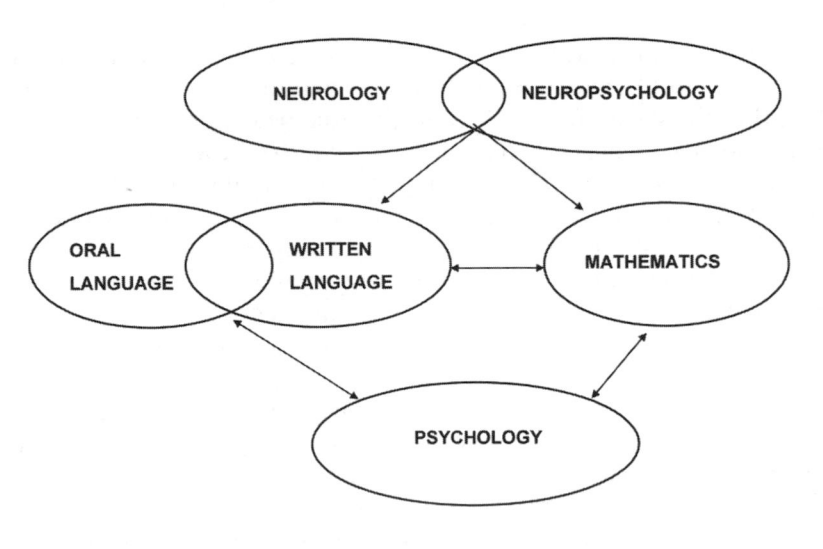

FIGURE 7.1. Schematic depiction of interrelationship among specialist evaluations in building a model of a child–world system.

in light of developmental challenges the child will encounter. Thus, current observations are used to predict potential later effects, within and across disciplines.

Since the evaluation is guided by developmental neuropsychological theory, the neurology and neuropsychology evaluations provide the conceptual core that establishes a fundamental brain–behavior hypothesis about the child's profile. The *neurological examination* includes a medical and developmental history, the classic neurological examination to assess potential neurological impairment, and an extended neurodevelopmental examination to assess motor and sensory signs that may corroborate the neuropsychological profile. The *neuropsychologist* describes the basic neurocognitive profile, including level of cognitive functioning, information-processing characteristics across materials, problem-solving strategies, and quality of the knowledge base. The test protocol samples from each of the major IQ indices, processing of complex visual and verbal material, as well as laboratory and observer reports of executive functioning. Close attention is paid to qualitative aspects of behavior (language quality; spontaneous comments; emotional, cognitive, and behavioral regulation; motivation; problem solving; social skills), enriching test interpretation.

Next the evaluation tracks manifestations of the neuropsychological profile in the context of language, communication, and academic skills. The *oral and written language evaluation* samples elements of oral language as well as reading and writing. Because of the intimate relationship between oral and written language, the two are evaluated in tandem. Difficulty understanding or formulating oral language will be reflected in reading and especially writing, manifest more prominently in complex academic tasks. Word decoding and recognition, reading comprehension, and reading rate are evaluated directly, with an estimate of competencies in relation to grade-level placement. Spelling and writing conventions (e.g., punctuation, sentence structure) as well as handwriting are important foundations that are assessed by a brief writing sample. Oral rehearsal of the writing sample provides insight into the impact of oral language on writing. The *mathematics evaluation* also uses curriculum-referenced materials to sample various aspects of mathematics knowledge and problem-solving behaviors, including developmental foundations, number concepts, arithmetic operations, geometry, applications to real-world problems, and mathematics problem-solving style. The academic evaluators pay particular attention to the neuropsychological profile and how it may or may not be manifest in the academic arena, as well as to prediction of future challenges in view of the developmental and curricular tasks that the child will confront. By the same token, particulars of academic performance can serve as grist for the neuropsychologist's mill.

Finally, the psychology evaluation assesses psychosocial functioning in the home and at school, especially self-efficacy and self-esteem, affect regulation, and social skills. Children with learning problems often experience erosion of self-efficacy and self-esteem, which can lead to depression and anxiety, a potential developmental cascade. Children who are well behaved in school may exhibit significant behavioral problems at home; they manage their stress with great effort all day, but then release it at home. Family stressors are also important; a child with vulnerabilities to learning disorders can be further derailed if he or she also needs to process a stressful life event such as a family illness or divorce. Genetic predispositions for psychiatric conditions (e.g., anxiety disorder) and other factors are also considered. Moreover, on a neuropsychological basis, as indicated above, many children with learning problems also have trouble learning social skills. This difficulty can further contribute to school-related anxiety and distress, as the child must navigate treacherous peer interactions in addition to academic challenges. The psychology examination also delineates protective factors and sources of resiliency, which can have an important bearing on school functioning. Whereas some children may be highly sensitive to failure or school struggles, others may be more resilient, based on either internal or external factors. Children who are better adjusted and feel understood and supported are more available for instruction.

THE CASE OF ALEXANDER AND BENJAMIN

Well, I think there's maybe one teacher who knows the difference of
who's who. I think many, many times they confused the two of them.
—ALEXANDER AND BENJAMIN'S DAD

Genetic factors clearly play an important role in reading problems; identical twins, who share all their genetic material, are much more similar in their reading abilities than are fraternal twins, who share only half. But developmental processes can also play a powerful role, potentially modifying gene expression at all levels of development. The complex interplay between genetic and experiential influences can emerge clearly when we meet identical twins as people rather than statistics, focusing on the whole child rather than the discrete skill. Identical twins, who as a group show great similarities statistically, can also display striking differences at an individual level. Twins, therefore, serve not only to highlight the powerful role of genes but, equally important, the impressive contribution of developmental processes. Understanding these phenomena in identical twins can inform a more general understanding of the role of developmental processes in outcomes. Moreover, following Bronfenbrenner, these biological processes are best understood in the *broadest social context*, which will inevitably have a material impact on development.

History

Alexander and Benjamin are identical twins who presented for clinical evaluation at the end of their fifth-grade year. They live in an exurban community of working people that, while certainly not impoverished, has significant economic limitations. Median household income in the town is roughly $65,000, with 34% of adult heads of household holding professional or management jobs. The twins' parents are vocational high school graduates. Their father works as a manager for a large supermarket chain while their mother stays at home with the children.

In the twins' middle school, roughly 13% of students are entitled to free or reduced-price lunch. In terms of state-mandated testing, 70% of fifth graders achieve scores in the proficient range or higher in English and language arts but only 48% for mathematics. Although the community is stable, the tax base is modest and school resources are tight. These resource limitations would play a dramatic role in the boys' developmental course.

The twins were delivered at 35 weeks gestational age via cesarean section because Benjamin was experiencing placental insufficiency.

Alexander was Twin A, the first twin delivered, weighing 6 pounds, 12 ounces; Benjamin, weighing only 5 pounds, 8 ounces, was Twin B. Thus, at birth they had already had quite different experiences, their weights differing by more than a pound. Nonetheless, both boys were vigorous at birth. Alexander initially suffered from some mild lung problems, but was discharged from the hospital on day 7. Benjamin was readmitted to the hospital a week after birth for failure to thrive, but soon recovered. There were no concerns about language development or motor milestones.

As toddlers, the boys had mildly elevated lead levels, but the family moved and instituted dietary controls, and the levels returned to normal without treatment. Benjamin also had multiple ear infections, requiring pressure-equalizing tubes and removal of his adenoids. The family history is positive for learning disabilities as well as autoimmune disorders. Although both boys were born healthy without major medical problems, Benjamin's prenatal environment had been suboptimal and he also had a history of ear infections, which may affect language development. Each had modest perinatal problems, and both had comparable environmental exposures.

Although both boys were noted to have learning problems, Benjamin had the more concerning history. The boys attended Head Start and did well but entered kindergarten with Title I support for academics. By the fourth grade, Benjamin's academic problems had become very concerning. He did well in math but lagged in reading. Because of his problems, the school administered testing, which documented a Full Scale IQ of 110. Although no psychoeducational testing was done, Benjamin's scores on group testing early in the fifth grade were troubling, with reading and math skills at only the third-grade level. A standardized math test late in the fifth grade, however, indicated mid-sixth-grade skills. His scores on the state testing in English and language arts were in the "needs improvement" range. The school psychologist was concerned about poor sleep hygiene and suggested that their mother put them to bed earlier (they typically slept from 9:00 P.M. until 6:00 A.M.).

Benjamin's fifth-grade teacher reported that he showed little or no affect in school and had difficulty working with other children. He was said to be very artistic, but his work habits were "inconsistent," and he was at times "passive–aggressive." The teacher was concerned about his lack of motivation and his preoccupation with drawing, which she felt interfered with his completing his work. She said he often shut out what was going on around him and "lacked the social skills to succeed in school," having been sent to the office on a number of occasions for aggressive behavior. Clearly, the teacher's attribution (and presumably that of others in the school) was that Benjamin's problems were primarily volitional and behavioral, not cognitive.

Although Alexander's picture was more favorable, his parents were also concerned about him. School testing in the fourth grade documented average IQ (Full Scale IQ 104), a bit lower than Benjamin's score. In contrast, however, his academic skills on the same group testing were at the mid-fourth-grade level early in the fifth grade, mildly delayed but not nearly as much as those of his brother. Also in contrast to his brother was his temperament. Whereas Benjamin was sensitive and easily stressed, Alexander was typically relaxed and sociable. His teacher commented: "Nothing seems to bother Alexander. He does not appear to be upset when he does not meet success." Like his brother, Alexander was a good artist, but unlike his brother, he was said by his teacher to have strong interpersonal skills. Again, however, she focused on a behavioral attribution to explain his academic problems, not a cognitive one.

Although they qualified for Title I support through the fourth grade, that program was no longer available in middle school, and neither had qualified for special education based on the school testing. Yet Benjamin was obviously in considerable distress. His parents frequently received notes from school that he was failing, and he would spend hours on homework. Moreover, he was exhibiting "meltdowns" at home, refusing to do homework. The behavioral problems at school were escalating, often triggered by bullying. Benjamin's mother observed that he would misinterpret cues, overreacting and becoming aggressive, perhaps fueled by his academic frustration.

Alexander also had difficulty with the fifth-grade curriculum. His teacher reported that he would often stare out the window. He too was beginning to exhibit meltdowns with increased homework, possibly reflecting some contagion from his more severely affected brother. Behavioral similarities between twins of course have genetic bases. But they can also reflect their intimate connection and opportunities for modeling and imitation, not to mention the tendency of others to view them as a unit. Frustrated by the school's unwillingness to acknowledge their problems and concerned about their children, the family sought independent evaluations. In order to minimize potential for confusing the boys, the evaluations were carried out 3 months apart.

Testing and Observation

Although the boys were hard to distinguish physically, their personalities were indeed distinct. Whereas Benjamin was shy and quiet, Alexander had an assured manner and when cognitively challenged would often

try to distract with his charm rather than commit effort. Their performances were indeed similar in many ways, but there were also substantial differences. The findings are summarized in Figure 7.2 according to
the schematic illustrated in Figure 7.1.

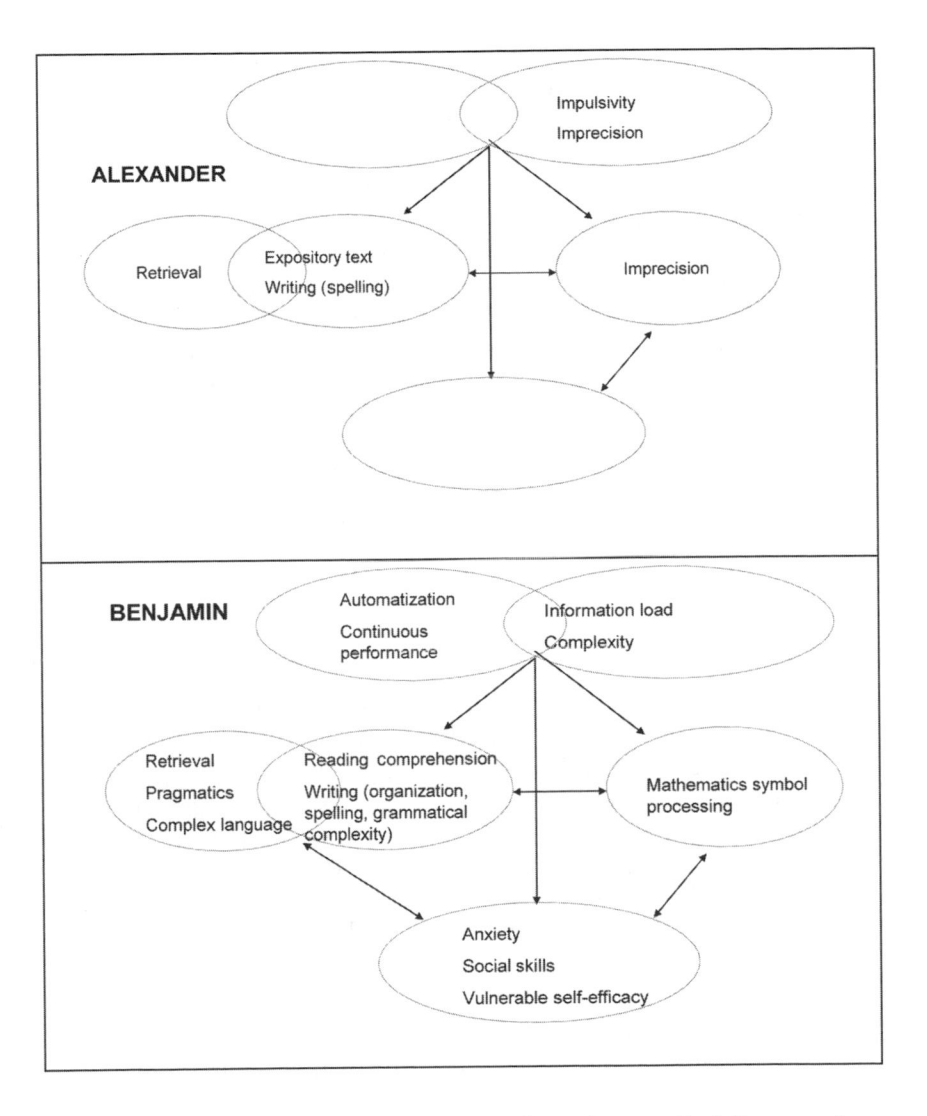

FIGURE 7.2. Schematic depiction of findings from the interdisciplinary evaluations of Alexander and Benjamin. Labels indicate areas of difficulty. Strengths
are not included here for simplicity of presentation.

Neurology

Benjamin, but not Alexander, had prominent difficulties on the extended neurodevelopmental component of the examination, especially on rapid automatized naming (RAN) (Denckla & Rudel, 1976). As was described in Chapter 5, the RAN is a deceptively simple task on which the child is asked to read off an array of stimuli (e.g., letters, numbers, colors, pictures of objects) displayed in rows on a card and repeated in a random order. Slow automatized naming is prevalent in children with learning problems, including, but by no means limited to, reading problems (Waber, Wolff, et al., 2000). Benjamin's automatized naming was exceedingly slow, especially for letters (4 *SD*s below the mean), consistent with high risk for learning problems of all sorts, but especially reading, because the letters condition was particularly slow (Waber, Wolff, et al., 2000; Wolf & Bowers, 1999). He also had trouble with a continuous performance test, often indicative of an attention disorder but, equally possible, of difficulty processing rapidly presented information. Structured ADHD questionnaires indicated that Benjamin had inattention symptoms in the clinical range, but only on the teacher version. The parent report did not reach clinical levels. For Alexander, neither the parents nor the teacher noted an elevation of symptoms. *Thus, Benjamin was at far greater neurodevelopmental risk than Alexander.*

Neuropsychology

Cognitive test scores are displayed in Table 7.1. There are many similarities, consistent with the typically high correlation of ability scores between identical twins. Yet there are also functionally salient differences. Benjamin had far more difficulty than his brother managing complex language. For example, the boys were asked to listen to and repeat brief narrative passages from the Children's Memory Scale (CMS) Stories subtest (Cohen, 1997). The first story is about two girls who witness a robbery and then provide information leading to the apprehension of the criminals. This was Alexander's repetition:

> "Lisa and Melissa were walking past the grocery store when these two men walked out of the store with a bag of money and hopped into a brown car and got away was out of there very fast. The police came and Eleesa told them the color of the car and Meleesa told there was a short guy and a tall guy and when they were there at the right moment at the right time the two criminals dudes were caught a month later."

TABLE 7.1. Representative Neuropsychological, Achievement, and Behavioral Rating Scores for Alexander and Benjamin

	Alexander	Benjamin
WISC-IV (scaled score)		
Information	10	8
Vocabulary	11	10
Digit Span	8	14
Coding	10	9
Block Design	10	11
Rey–Osterrieth Complex Figure		
Copy Organization	25%ile	75%ile
Immediate Recall Organization	50%ile	50%ile
Immediate Recall Errors	> 10%ile	< 10%ile
Delayed Recall Organization	10%ile	50%ile
Delayed Recall Errors	> 10%ile	< 10%ile
CMS Stories (scaled score)		
Immediate	11	9
Delayed	10	8
Delayed Recognition	12	9
D-KEFS Color–Word Interference (scaled score)		
Color	10	9
Word	8	10
Interference	10	2
Interference Errors	2	1

	Parent	Teacher	Parent	Teacher
Behavioral Rating Inventory of Executive Functions (*t*-score)				
Behavioral Regulation Index	60	51	55	56
Metacognitive Index	67	67	58	72

	Alexander	Benjamin
Wechsler Individual Achievement Test— Word Reading (standard score)	104	102
Qualitative Reading Inventory–4 Comprehension	Instructional grade 6 (narrative); grade 5 (expository)	Instructional grade 3
Mathematics Diagnostic and Prescriptive Inventory	Late 5	Late 5/early 6
Behavior Assessment System for Children	Within normal limits (parent and teacher)	At risk: Attention (parent and teacher); Learning, Adaptive Skills (teacher only)

Although imprecise and distorted in places, Alexander's repetition preserves much of the original narrative and elaborated detail, suggesting that his fundamental language capacities are adequately developed, as reflected in his score. By contrast, Benjamin's immediate repetition was as follows:

> "Lisa and her sister were on their way to the grocery store when two men jumped in front of them with a money bag. They jumped into the car and went away. Because Lisa and her sister were in the right place the men were caught a month later."

Although Benjamin captures the basic gist, his repetition is sparse, providing little detail, and distorted (in the story, the girls were not sisters, and they were headed to school, not the grocery store). The highly detailed language was overwhelming for him from the standpoint of both language processing and information load.

Benjamin, however, outperformed Alexander significantly on the WISC-IV Digit Span subtest (Wechsler, 2003), on which they were to repeat strings of random digits in the forward and then backward order, possibly because he worked hard to use his rote memory without needing to process complex language. Alexander, who was more easygoing, might have invested less effort. Yet Benjamin was the boy whom the teachers viewed as lacking motivation and failing to invest effort!

The boys' performance on the Rey–Osterrieth Complex Figure Test (Bernstein & Waber, 1996), on which they were asked to copy and then draw from memory a complex geometric design, was remarkably similar (Figure 7.3), especially considering that they were evaluated nearly 3 months apart and could not plausibly have communicated their solutions. The ROCF is a complicated geometric design that the child copies and then draws from memory. Children with learning problems can tend to focus on the appended details rather than on the logical geometric structure of the figure. Although children typically produce better organized copies of the figure as they get older, children referred for learning problems, as a group, level off at the 8- to 9-year level without further gains (Waber & Bernstein, 1995).

Benjamin again worked diligently; he produced a nice copy of the complex figure by working in an incremental part-by-part fashion. Alexander impulsively conflated the cross at the bottom of the design with the bottom side of the rectangle. Remarkably, both made the same error in copying the small box embedded in the left side of the figure, adding a vertical line to the middle of the box. Moreover, their recall productions were alike, capturing the overall shape but failing to integrate the two sides, highlighting their difficulty managing complex information,

ALEXANDER   **BENJAMIN**

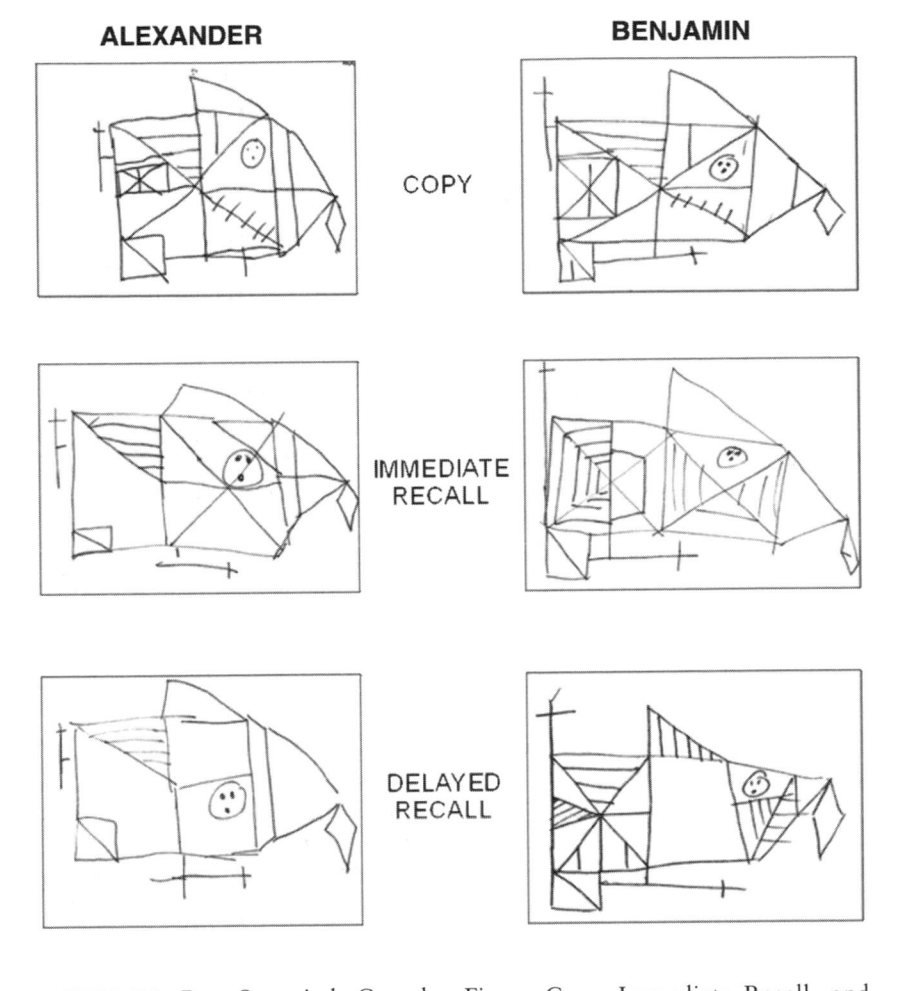

COPY

IMMEDIATE
RECALL

DELAYED
RECALL

FIGURE 7.3. Rey–Osterrieth Complex Figure Copy, Immediate Recall, and Delayed Recall productions for Alexander and Benjamin.

especially if it is unfamiliar and cannot be anchored in their prior knowledge. Whereas Alexander displaces the diagonals to the right, Benjamin replicates them on both sides, adding lines perseveratively to fill the space. Benjamin's delayed recall preserves the organizational structure but contains significantly more distortion. Alexander preserves the overall configuration but his organization score is low because he forgets the main diagonals. Benjamin's production indicates how very confused details can become in his memory, just as they did on the stories. Despite confusing details, however, Benjamin's productions are actually well organized, reminiscent of his ability to extract basic themes from the stories. His confusion is reflected in the Error score (which quantifies distortions), which is in the impaired range, whereas Alexander's is within normal limits.

The Delis–Kaplan Executive Function System (D-KEFS) Color–Word Interference Test is a version of the Stroop test, a classic psychological measure of cognitive control, or inhibition (Delis, Kaplan, & Kramer, 2001). The child first names a random array of color patches, then reads a comparable field of color names, and finally must name the ink color of a color name printed in conflicting color ink (e.g., the correct response for the word *red* written in green ink would be *green*). Both boys performed well on the simple Color and Word conditions, but their performance deteriorated with the increased demands of the Interference condition, indicating their susceptibility to cognitive dysregulation with information load. Alexander maintained his speed but made many errors, consistent with his carefree demeanor and at times impulsive approach. Benjamin, however, characteristically slowed down substantially yet made even more errors, indicating his significantly greater vulnerability to information-processing load, as the neurology examination had forecast. This pattern was consistent with his very slow automatized naming, cluttering of details on the Rey–Osterrieth Complex Figure recall, and loss and distortion of information on story repetition, as well as his poor showing on the continuous performance task. He was diligent and attended well, yet simply could not keep up.

Although the boys showed remarkable similarities and both have legitimate sources of school difficulties, *Benjamin clearly exhibited more substantial risk, consistent with their school performance and with the neurology examination.* These neuropsychological profiles would be manifested in their academic performances.

Oral and Written Language

Not surprisingly, the boys performed differently on their oral and written language evaluation. Benjamin made clear his displeasure with academic pursuits. He had trouble with word retrieval as well as with understanding and using higher-order language. Pragmatically, he did not consistently appreciate the thrust and intention of what others were saying, consistent with his reticent social presentation and with his mother's theory that his aggression stemmed in part from difficulty interpreting social cues.

In his reading, Benjamin could, with effort, decode a word list at his grade placement, but his comprehension was estimated at only the third-grade level (mirroring his strength in simple digit repetition and weakness in the more linguistically complex story repetition). Again, he had difficulty integrating cues and context to make sense of the text, becoming flooded with the information. He also had difficulty with the higher-order language demands of comprehension.

As alluded to earlier, many children who can diligently respond to evidence-based interventions focused on phonics and decoding remain functionally delayed because their comprehension, which depends on higher-order language competence, continues to lag and/or they fail to acquire fluency (or automaticity). Benjamin was such a person. His limitations in higher-order language competence as well as information processing and automaticity substantially constrained his ability to derive meaning from text at the level of his placement, despite his ability to decode.

Alexander had mild word retrieval problems, but in contrast to his brother, was adept at using context to facilitate his language comprehension, just as he more adeptly appraised the social context. His word recognition skills were nearly identical to his brother's. Were we to focus on single-word reading, a typical benchmark, the correlation between these twins would indeed be very high. Yet Alexander's comprehension was substantially better, in line with his oral language and the quality of his information processing. He read competently in sixth-grade narrative text, but only at a frustration level in expository material, indicative of his risk in the content curriculum at his placement. His writing, although better than Benjamin's, still reflected difficulty with organization and integration. Importantly, whereas Benjamin was simply unprepared to engage with the curriculum at the sixth-grade level, Alexander would be able to manage with in-class support and accommodations.

Not surprisingly, Benjamin's writing was also more significantly delayed. The grammatical structures were simple, consisting of subject–verb sentences sometimes joined by *and*. The content was disorganized and did not consistently make sense, and there were numerous spelling errors, often homophonic (e.g., *I* for *eye*, *there* for *they're*). Alexander's writing, although also disorganized, used more complex grammatical forms, such as subordinate clauses, and the spelling errors reflected imprecision (e.g., *favorit* for *favorite*, *thats* for *that's*), consistent with the rest of his work.

Mathematics

Both boys did well in math, Benjamin surprisingly so, given his struggles with reading and information processing, but their cognitive profiles emerged here as well. Benjamin's skills were at the late fifth to early sixth-grade level, with strengths in broad perspectives and logical problem solving, like his performance on the Rey figure. His processing of the symbolic components of math, however, was inefficient, cluttered with numerous restarts and repairs, again reflecting his general cognitive profile. Alexander shifted between global and linear strategies, but his skills were also appropriate for his placement. Consistent with his impulsive style, his efforts could be compromised by imprecision.

Psychology

Not surprisingly, Benjamin was the more vulnerable boy emotionally. He was a worrier, would avoid challenging tasks in school, and struggled socially, all of which could be referred to his cognitive profile. Although his self-esteem and self-efficacy remained intact, they were clearly vulnerable to erosion. Alexander, in contrast, appeared well adjusted and well behaved, with secure self-esteem.

Diagnosis: The Child–World Interaction

These identical twins exhibited many similarities in their test scores: their IQs were comparable, as was their single-word reading ability; they were more skilled at math than reading; they had word retrieval problems; and their drawings of the Rey complex figure were remarkably alike. But they also differed in ways that were highly relevant for their functional adaptation and that shaped the school's response to them: Their personalities and cognitive styles were different; they differed in their ability to use verbal and social contexts and to manage higher-order language; their functional reading and writing skills were very different, as was their information processing and vulnerability to information load. These similarities and differences are reflected in the summary diagnostic formulations from the evaluations, excerpted below:

Alexander

"Alexander is an 11-year-old rising sixth grader of average cognitive potential who can be vulnerable to details and information load, leading to inefficiency and imprecision, as well as difficulty integrating details into more coherent frameworks that could render his learning easier. These issues emerge most prominently in his comprehension of expository texts and in his written expression. He has learned avoidant strategies, and when overwhelmed, at least in this evaluation, he engaged socially and tried to distract with his charm. In the academic domain, his skills are solidly at grade level in mathematics, but he can struggle with reading grade level expository text and especially with writing. This is referable to his cognitive profile, which renders him at risk in material that is more complex, such that his basic skills, such as spelling, can break down in the context of the more complicated demands of writing. Psychologically, Alexander is well adjusted and remains confident despite his learning challenges, with good self-esteem."

Benjamin

"Benjamin is an 11-year-old ending fifth grader of average cognitive potential with a prominent learning disability and potentially a primary disorder of attention. Benjamin is basically well motivated, but his efforts are significantly undermined by his massive difficulty integrating information, his difficulty making use of context, and his significantly diminished automaticity and output. Because of these issues, he needs to work extremely hard to monitor himself and self-correct, often in the context of broader confusion, and the ensuing frustration is contributing to an emergent lack of investment in academics. His profile is affecting him most prominently in oral and written language, as well as in social skills development and application, and he cannot demonstrate his competencies in the school setting. His oral and written language skills, in particular, are significantly delayed (no more than third-grade skills at the end of the fifth grade), and he will be unable to manage the sixth-grade curriculum with these skills, *which is likely to trigger further disengagement and possibly escalating behavioral issues* [emphasis added]. Mathematics is better preserved, at grade level, and he can demonstrate some impressive logical problem-solving skills. There is also some suggestion from our findings that Benjamin meets criteria for an attention disorder (ADHD, inattentive subtype), but it is difficult to discern at this point how much of that is secondary to his struggles with information processing and output and the resulting disengagement and frustration."

Recommendations

The recommendations flowed directly from the diagnostic formulation. Since the primary goal is to improve the child's contextual adaptation, the recommendations are directed toward better aligning the child's profile and the environmental support and demands, thereby reducing distress and facilitating effective progress. Importantly, the recommendations are geared toward the whole child, not just specific skills. Following from the diagnostic formulations, the recommendations for the two boys were quite different. Benjamin's profile called for more substantial intervention:

1. The school should develop a comprehensive individualized education plan (IEP) to feature an integrated oral and written language program, with input from both a speech–language pathologist and a written language specialist. *[Benjamin's reading comprehension and writing, as well as his ability to integrate details contextually, especially in higher-order language, were significantly diminished. His functional reading would be associated with his language development and thus should be addressed in an integrated way. Single-word reading was not the issue and thus not a primary focus.]*

2. As Benjamin enters the sixth grade in the fall, the school team should meet early in the year to review the reports and develop an education plan for providing accommodations and supports across subject areas. *[In middle school the potential for fragmentation is great, as teachers focus on content areas rather than on the child's development. Consistent approaches and especially a consistent model of attribution, more accurate than the prevailing attributions of "lack of motivation" or "behavior problem," would be essential to inform accommodations and to facilitate Benjamin's positive functioning in school.]*

3. Because of his oral and written language compromise, Benjamin would need substantial adaptations across content areas (science, social studies, literature) as well as in terms of structuring tasks for him and integrating the development of metacognitive skills throughout the curriculum. Emphasis should be placed on the quality of his performance, rather than quantity, with accommodations to provide access to content material commensurate with his cognitive level, rather than at the level of his written language skills. *[Especially at the upper-elementary and middle-school levels, teachers may fail to appreciate that a child with compromised language skills will not be able to participate in content-area curricula, despite adequate cognitive competency. This can make school more frustrating or boring, as the choices are either to subject the child to unrealistic production demands, or to gear the conceptual level of instruction to the child's oral and written language, well below the potential for conceptual appreciation and thus interest and engagement.]*

4. Benjamin would benefit from curriculum-based social skills training. He would also benefit from a designated counselor or faculty member to help him manage his frustration and behavior in a constructive fashion. *[Benjamin's diminished appreciation of social cues, which can lead to misinterpretation, combined with his high level of academic frustration, have triggered some of his behavior problems, which will*

intensify and become a more "entrenched" part of his persona if his academic and psychosocial domains do not improve. He will need targeted psychosocial support to remain profitably engaged in academics and not become coded by teachers as a "behavior problem."]

5. Since the ADHD diagnosis was uncertain, medication should be considered only after Benjamin has had the benefit of an appropriate educational program. *[Although a child may exhibit symptoms that meet criteria for ADHD, these behaviors, especially inattentive symptoms, can be secondary to other cognitive issues, often higher-order language difficulties. Medication should be considered only after an appropriate educational plan is implemented, because the behaviors may not represent ADHD.]*

6. Benjamin's competencies in math, sports, and other extracurricular interests should be celebrated to buoy his confidence and self-esteem. *[It is easy to become so preoccupied with deficits that strengths and competencies are not recognized. Yet the competencies support the child emotionally through frustration and will ultimately be the basis for successful adult adaptation. Competencies, therefore, need to be attended to in equal measure.]*

The recommendations for Alexander were modest, in keeping with the narrower scope of the findings. Instead of an IEP, monitoring and accommodations were recommended but no direct services. Among the suggested accommodations was judicious adjustment of demands so that Alexander would not become overwhelmed by information load, as well as metacognitive supports throughout the curriculum.

Another recommendation was that teachers should be careful not to confuse the learning profiles of the two boys, and that they should help Alexander to appreciate his potential and to use it more effectively. A meeting between the parents and the teaching team early in the year to review the reports, as well as a point person in school with whom they could communicate and review school performance and homework compliance, would be helpful as well.

What Happened?

Midway through the seventh grade, a year and half after the boys had been evaluated, the parents reported that the assessments had been helpful for them, most importantly because a team of experts had corroborated their own perceptions. They understood better that, as they had suspected, Benjamin's problems were more significant than Alexander's. They became more aware of Alexander's avoidant strategies when he was challenged academically, but also that some of his challenges were legitimate and not simply due to lack of will. Although the parents had insisted for some time that their children had learning problems, the school had put them off. The parents had felt that school personnel talked down to them because they did not have sophisticated educational backgrounds. Now the evaluations had given them confidence. Nonetheless, the school had dismissed the reports, insisting that their own testing (only an IQ test) had not corroborated these needs. Although they did make some informal recommendations, their content did not appear to recognize the distinction between the boys.

The boys entered the sixth grade without any meaningful change in their educational programs. They were on separate teams, meaning that they had different teachers and different homework. For Benjamin in particular, the lack of academic support was a major emotional stressor, as the evaluation had predicted. He struggled through the fall term, becoming increasingly withdrawn and preoccupied with doodling. By the February vacation, Benjamin had 28 incomplete assignments, and the family spent the entire vacation helping him to catch up, as well as helping Alexander, who also had some incomplete assignments. Benjamin was very sad and would break down screaming that he had too much schoolwork and stress. With an attorney's help, individualized education plans were finally developed for the boys by the end of the sixth grade. Curiously, the plans called for modified homework for *Alexander*, not Benjamin. In any event, the school's response bore little relation to the extensive reports.

In the seventh grade Benjamin was placed in a "developmental reading" class with 20 students, including a number of youngsters with significant behavior problems, and one teacher. By then, Benjamin himself was apparently viewed primarily as a behavior problem because of his aggressive outbursts. In any event, this class was not the intensive integrated oral and written language program that had been recommended. Benjamin was, however, given the opportunity to attend an elective special needs class of 20 students instead of study hall. Promised classroom modifications did not occur. Without an adequate program, Benjamin predictably continued to decline academically and emotionally, a typical developmental cascade. Midway through the seventh grade, he had failed English and was now beginning to fail math as well. His parents observed that his aggressive episodes seemed to track his academic stress. When he caught up with his work, the aggression would diminish, but as he again fell behind, it would escalate and he would become more emotionally withdrawn, unfortunately confirming the predictions of the evaluation.

Despite their highly contentious interactions with the school, the parents believed that the school's attitudes and responses toward their concerns were not malevolent, but driven by a significant lack of resources. This situation trapped everyone, making the parent–school interaction a battleground rather than a collaboration. They did not, for example, report that other children were receiving services denied to their children; rather, they believed that the resources were simply unavailable. The special education staff were well intended but were themselves captive to the same limitations. Nevertheless, as parents, they felt compelled to continue to advocate for their children. They also had to become intimately involved, on a daily basis, with monitoring and supporting their children's academics, like so many parents of children with learning problems.

The story illustrates another important point. A twinship, especially identical twins, is not only of major biological consequence, but also exerts powerful experiential influences. Although the boys were on separate sixth-grade teams, in the seventh grade their parents requested the same team because they needed so much support from home. It was simply unsupportable to have them on different teams. Yet because of their placement, teachers more easily confused the boys and their academic needs.

Indeed, running through the history is the difficulty that adults have had distinguishing them, especially since they appear physically identical. By rights, Alexander should be much less distressed, but he is also experiencing genuine school-related distress. Since the boys are so emotionally and experientially connected, Alexander may internalize Benjamin's distress and perhaps struggle with school more than he needs to.

For the school, especially with the two boys on the same team, distinguishing them is a significant challenge, and this confusion can work to the detriment of both. According the twins' father, "I think maybe there's one teacher who knows the difference of who's who. I think many times they confuse the two of them, like when there's a discipline, who they told has an assignment or whatever ... because they've brought stuff up at meetings and we're like, what's he talking about? Oh, we're sorry, this is the other one." At one point, Alexander was taken out of class for reading help, and the parents were told that Benjamin was not eligible.

Even the parents, who clearly distinguish the boys and appreciate their many differences, frequently have trouble talking about them separately. They also struggle with managing the differences between the two boys. For example, when Alexander does well academically, they are reluctant to praise him lest Benjamin, who worked just as hard in the same curriculum, become even more discouraged. Alexander is then less motivated to invest effort. In these circumstances, it is easy to see how twins can come to resemble one another more, despite their differences, and how Alexander could "catch" Benjamin's distress. Thus, environmental forces can function to heighten their similarities along with their genetics.

Commentary: The Developmental Perspective

As promised, twins have much to teach us about the developmental perspective. They reinforce the principle that *because of the indistinct boundaries between gene, brain, and environment, appearances of innateness should be questioned*. Despite their similarities, there were significant differences at a fundamental neurodevelopmental level, including, importantly, their temperaments and ultimately their personalities. Moreover, aspects of their experience, including their being twins, served not only to effect differences but to enhance similarities.

Especially important for these boys was the *larger system, involving both proximal (family and school) and distal (government, society) influences*. The developmental impact of the broader context for these boys cannot be overemphasized. Their school district—perhaps because of economic limitations, perhaps because of the school culture—seemed to commit limited resources to special education. Especially troubling, the culture of special education appeared to focus almost entirely on the gatekeeper function, with relatively less investment in the child's well-being. Although it was clear from the evaluations what each boy needed to repair the dysfunctional interaction in the child–world system, virtually no steps were taken to make this happen or even to acknowledge that there was a legitimate problem, especially for Benjamin.

The conflicting attributions of the family and school were critical. Because of his social skills problems and aggressive outbursts, Benjamin acquired a reputation as a behavior problem, which had become entrenched as his primary persona. The school seemed unable or unwilling to entertain the alternative, or perhaps additional, attribution supported in great detail by data from the evaluation. Benjamin was not a "bad actor"; he was a child with a language-based learning disability for whom school had become significantly frustrating and distressing and who responded with aggression. Nevertheless, the school focused on that aspect of his presentation and seemed frustrated that the parents were unable to control Benjamin. Sadly, considerable positive change could have been achieved at little financial cost had the school been willing to reframe their understanding of the boys. In Benjamin's case, the reframing would have been inadequate without direct services, but it could at least have modified the character of their day-to-day management of him in important ways. Since the school evaluation was largely about allocating scarce resources, however, being open to reframing would also have obliged them to provide resources. Their failure to do so, whatever their reason, further contributed to Benjamin's downward cascade, and by extension, to Alexander's. Unfortunately, in this case, the child–world system predictably became more, rather than less, dysfunctional over time, as the parents and school became further enmeshed in their struggle rather than channeling their resources toward solving the problem.

Chapter 8

An Adequate Achiever with Learning Problems

With a learning disability, it's like you want the cure for
the disease ... like if we could find the exact problem, then
maybe we could find the cure, which is not really the case.
—ANDREW'S MOTHER

For many children who struggle with learning problems, documenting a bona fide "specific learning disability" is not a black-and-white undertaking, but falls in a gray zone. When children continue to struggle yet manage to achieve adequate scores on all the psychoeducational testing, diagnosis can be elusive. These children can prove especially confounding for parents who struggle to understand their child's problems in relation to the available diagnostic "bins" (e.g., dyslexia, ADD, nonverbal learning disability). Sometimes everyone suspects there is a problem, but no one can "put a finger on it." The research described in Chapter 5 documented the basic information-processing profiles of these children. In this chapter we meet one such boy.

THE CASE OF ANDREW

History

Andrew, a fifth grader, lives with his mother, father, 13-year-old sister (who does well in school), and 4-year-old brother. His mother holds a master's degree in computer science and works part-time from home. His father, a college graduate, is a manager in a transportation company. The family lives in an affluent suburban town where the median income is roughly $100,000. Most heads of household hold managerial or professional jobs, and 68% hold graduate degrees. Standards for academic achievement are high. On the state-mandated testing, 85% of Andrew's fifth-grade peers scored in the proficient to advanced range in both English/language arts and mathematics. Ninety percent of high school graduates attend 4-year colleges. The culture of both the classroom and the community at large, therefore, is competitive, with high expectations for achievement.

Developmentally, Andrew was somewhat late to talk, using only 10 words by his second birthday. His comprehension was good, however, and connected speech emerged shortly after he turned 2, so early intervention was not needed. Nevertheless, this delay was developmental evidence of a vulnerability in the language system. He had recurrent ear infections, eventually resulting in the placement of tubes. He also had problems in his fine motor development, another marker of developmental risk. At nearly 11 years old, he was slow to tie his shoes and had trouble with Velcro closures on jackets. In contrast, his gross motor development was advanced, and he excelled athletically, a source of pride and satisfaction for him.

As early as preschool, Andrew's educational career was intermittently punctuated by concerns on the part of his teachers and parents, but these concerns were never severe and consistent enough to merit formal special education identification. Andrew spent 2 years in preschool and did well, but midway through the second year the teacher suggested that he might not be ready for kindergarten. By April, he had rallied sufficiently to go on to kindergarten. During that year, the teacher again expressed concern, but by the end of the year, he had made sufficient progress to enter first grade. He had a strict teacher that year, which was hard on him because he was shy and eager to please, but he could not always do so easily. Since his reading was progressing slowly, he received help from a reading specialist, but he was not put on an IEP. In general, he just seemed to need a little more teacher direction. Toward the end of that year, the teacher yet again expressed concerns and suggested that perhaps Andrew should repeat the grade. School testing (Table 8.1) yielded scores that were all in the average range, basically unremarkable, and Andrew was deemed to have no special needs.

And so, doubts trailing in his wake, Andrew went to second grade, where he surprised everyone by doing well. The teacher's style worked well for him, and Andrew's parents hoped he had outgrown his problems. Yet in third grade, with a different teacher and more demanding work, the doubts returned. When his mother volunteered in Andrew's class, she saw that his writing was not up to that of peers.

TABLE 8.1. Representative Scores from Andrew's School Testing Completed in the First and Fourth Grades

	Grade 1	Grade 4
WISC-III Full Scale IQ	106	117
WIAT (percentile)		
Reading	32	55
Mathematics	50	87
Written Language	70	87
Oral Language	61	99
WRAML (percentile)		
Verbal Memory	45	66
Visual Memory	55	79
Learning Index	79	97
CELF-3 (percentile)		
Receptive	82	—
Expressive	61	—
Rey–Osterrieth Complex Figure (percentile)	—	50–75

Note. WISC-II, Wechsler Intelligence Scale for Children–III; WIAT, Wechsler Individual Achievement Test; WRAML, Wide Range Assessment of Memory and Learning; CELF-3, Clinical Evaluation of Language Fundamentals–3.

Andrew's parents were once again concerned. Since kindergarten, they had received the consistent (if inconsistently delivered) message that something was wrong, but never wrong enough, to merit special treatment. Testing had not identified a clear problem, and the only solution that had ever been offered was grade retention, which did not seem like a good one. With no apparent alternative in the public school, they thought private school might provide a better option by giving him the personal attention he seemed to need. In preparation for a possible application, Andrew took an IQ test, which documented strong competencies. This finding came as something of a surprise given his checkered history, and everyone wondered why his school performance was not better. Perhaps Andrew *did* have a learning disability.

Still frustrated and uncertain, but not yet ready to take him out of the neighborhood school, Andrew's parents sent him on to the fourth grade. The family again requested school testing, which once again found no basis for concern (Table 8.1). Indeed, in many areas, Andrew's performance was strong. Given his exemplary performance on the testing, the school still had no rationale to formally recognize his problems or provide him with extra support. Perhaps, they implied, in this high-pressure community, Andrew's parents were simply overly concerned.

Consistent in his inconsistency, Andrew did well, perhaps because of the sensitivity or style of the teacher. Despite his classroom success, however, Andrew's scores on state-mandated testing triggered the next alarm. In a town in which 85% of students score in the proficient to advanced range, indicating that the quality of the instruction is excellent, Andrew was less successful. His Mathematics score was only in the "needs improvement" range, and English/Language Arts barely reached "proficient."

Andrew's fifth-grade teacher expressed concern about his erratic test performance and wondered whether his problems were due to anxiety. She described him as a quiet, friendly boy who was generally attentive, always well behaved, and followed directions; he was respectful and participated appropriately in class. The teacher also reported that he had a good background of general knowledge, knew his math facts and operations, and did well with peers. She was concerned, however, that his poor test scores did not reflect his ability. Under pressure, he could forget to do even simple tasks that should have been easy for him. Asked to characterize Andrew's problems, his mother observed perceptively that he did not know how to be strategic in order to make things simpler for himself. "Whatever he sees or hears," she remarked, "he takes at face value."

This story is by no means unusual: the child for whom nagging questions persist, but whose profile is never sufficiently dramatic to meet standard criteria for specific learning disability. He thus never receives particular support or even formal acknowledgment, that is, *permission* for his problems, which in and of itself can often be therapeutic. Moreover, scores on well-respected psychoeducational tests consistently documented adequate competence. This situation was not the fault of the teachers, who had repeatedly raised concerns, and several rounds of competent testing had been conducted. Yet something was wrong—there was clearly dysfunction in the child–world system. Despite everyone's good intentions, there was simply no appropriate officially sanctioned box to contain Andrew's situation.

Andrew's parents sought independent evaluation during the fifth grade to find out, once and for all, whether their son had a learning disability. His history raised a series of hypotheses that would be systematically examined in the course of the evaluation:

- He had a bona fide learning disability that the testing had failed to detect.
- He had cognitive issues that undermined his academic performance but had been able to partially compensate for them.

- He had an anxiety disorder that interfered with his academic functioning.
- He was simply an average child living in an above-average world.

Testing and Observation

Figure 8.1 illustrates the results of the examination schematically.

Neurology

Although the extended neurodevelopmental examination was essentially normal, some motor maneuvers, such as hopping on one foot, were notably effortful. On the RAN test (Denckla & Rudel, 1976), Andrew performed slowly on symbolic items (Letters and Numbers) and even more slowly with alternating categories (Letters and Objects). The fact that symbols were more prominently affected suggests a neurodevelopmental risk for processing symbolic material; difficulty with alternating stimuli can signal problems with executive control and complexity. *These findings argued against several hypotheses: Andrew was not simply a child with average cognitive potential in an above-average world, nor were his problems solely attributable to test anxiety.*

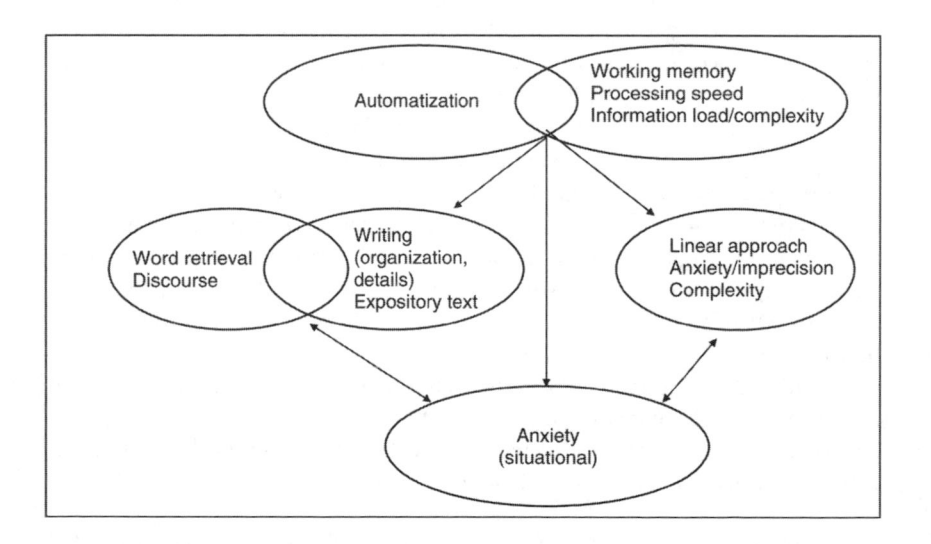

FIGURE 8.1. Schematic depiction of findings from the interdisciplinary evaluation of Andrew. Labels indicate areas of difficulty. Strengths not included here for simplicity of presentation.

Neuropsychology

Andrew's scores on selected WISC-IV subtests indicated very solid verbal knowledge and reasoning skills, but he performed more poorly on measures of *working memory* and *processing speed*—cognitive processes that are often depressed in children with learning problems (Table 8.2) and that are consistent with his diminished cognitive efficiency, as

TABLE 8.2. Representative Neuropsychological, Achievement, and Behavioral Scores for Andrew from Interdisciplinary Evaluation

WISC-IV (scaled score)		
Information	12	
Vocabulary	11	
Digit Span	7	
Coding	7	
Block Design	12	
Rey–Osterrieth Complex Figure		
Copy Organization	< 10%ile	
Immediate Recall Organization	25%ile	
Delayed Recall Organization	25%ile	
CMS Stories (scaled score)		
Immediate	14	
Delayed	16	
Delayed Recognition	12	
D-KEFS Color–Word Interference (scaled score)		
Color	12	
Word	10	
Interference	10	
Interference Errors	9	
	Parent	Teacher
Behavioral Rating Inventory of Executive Functions (*t*-score)		
Behavioral Regulation Index	38	54
Metacognitive Index	63	57
Wechsler Individual Achievement Test— Word Reading (standard score)	102	
Qualitative Reading Inventory–4— Comprehension	Grade 5 (expository); did not meet comprehension criteria	
Mathematics Diagnostic and Prescriptive Inventory	Late 5/early 6; linear, step-by-step style	
Behavior Assessment System for Children	Externalizing 32; Internalizing 47	

Note. WISC-IV, Wechsler Intelligence Scale for Children–IV; CMS, Children's Memory Scale; D-KEFS, Delis–Kaplan Executive Function System.

highlighted by the RAN. He worked at a slow deliberate pace and could become overwhelmed when he initially encountered material that he experienced as complicated and thus challenging. In these situations, he would adopt a rigidly linear, part-by-part strategy, without recognizing organizing frameworks and contexts at a more conceptual level. With extended exposure to the material or external structure, he was much more effective. His profile, nonetheless, would become increasingly intrusive in the middle school curriculum.

The cognitive profile was clearly reflected on the Rey–Osterrieth Complex Figure Test (Figure 8.2). In his copy, Andrew started with the

ANDREW

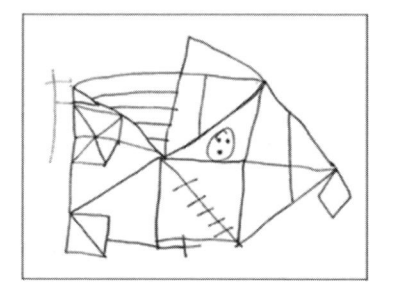

COPY

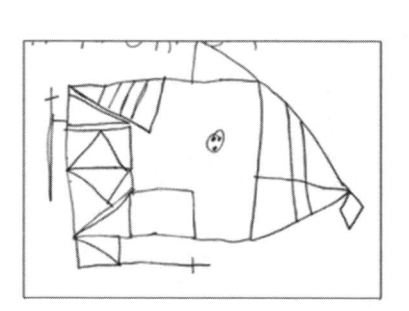

IMMEDIATE RECALL

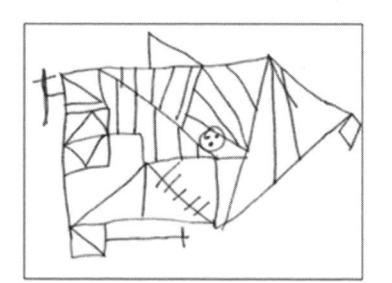

DELAYED
RECALL

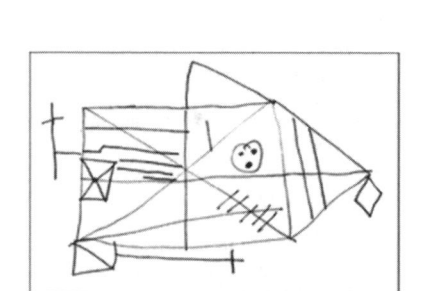

STRUCTURED
PRESENTATION
IMMEDIATE RECALL

FIGURE 8.2. Rey–Osterrieth Complex Figure, Copy, Immediate Recall, and Delayed Recall productions as well as Immediate Recall after structured presentation for Andrew.

first detail that captured his attention and then worked incrementally, without assigning greater importance to lines with more organizational significance. He approached each line at "face value," in his mother's terms, rather than assimilating it into a meaningful framework. Although he eventually did a nice job by using the model to guide him line by line, he worked hard to do so. Because he had not processed the figure as an organized whole, moreover, he missed an important structural element (a piece of the lower horizontal side; Figure 8.2, Copy), significantly lowering his score (< 10%ile), reminiscent of his teacher's concern about missing details. Andrew's difficulty with integrating the multiple elements into a coherent figure would typify his approach when he encountered more challenging academic tasks.

The immediate recall drawing indicates how Andrew had understood the complex design. As he copied it, he had apparently become aware of the basic rectangular shape, but not the logical organization of the figure or its details. He drew the rectangle and then entered several elements, but they were not integrated with the figure, and there was considerable empty space. On the delayed recall, he filled the space with repetitive lines, attempting to comply with the demand because he knew something was there.

At the end of the session, the Rey figure was presented again, this time in a structured format using transparent overlays, with the basic rectangle presented first and the external and then the internal details added incrementally (Figure 8.3) (Kirkwood, Weiler, Bernstein, Forbes, & Waber, 2001; Waber et al., 1994). With the benefit of this structure, Andrew immediately grasped the organization; even more encouraging, his memory production was nearly flawless (Figure 8.2). Thus, with modest external structure and redirection, he rallied and did quite well.

Andrew's performance highlighted his tendency to approach complex or unfamiliar materials not well anchored in his knowledge base at face value, as his mother so aptly observed, driven by salient details rather than actively extracting or inferring concepts and frameworks to anchor his efforts. Such difficulties can often be invisible to reliable psychoeducational instruments that typically present test items as discrete items. Yet they can have significant ecological implications, especially in middle school, when the curriculum anticipates an ability to apply skills and to manage more novel, abstract, and complex material. This characteristic is not uncommon among children referred for learning problems and is reminiscent of the interplay between the frontal and parietal regions, as suggested in Chapter 6. Because Andrew does not easily recognize underlying patterns (integration), he resorts to a diligent, *effortful*, piece-by-piece strategy that is inefficient and sometimes

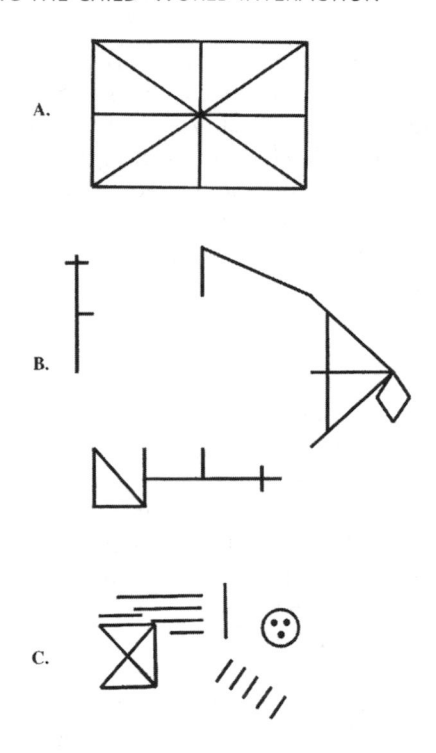

FIGURE 8.3. Structured presentation of Rey–Osterrieth Complex Figure. Child copies rectangle (A), then outer detail (B) is added with clear acetate overlay and child is to copy, and finally inner details are added (C). After copying design in this structured format, child is asked to draw again from memory. From Kirkwood, Weiler, Bernstein, Forbes, and Waber (2001). Copyright 2001 by Taylor & Francis. Reprinted by permission.

ineffective, undermining his executive functioning. The structured presentation, by supporting the integrative component of the task, greatly enhanced its execution. Once he understood the pattern, his effort was greatly reduced and the organization of the figure was excellent.

Like the neurological examination, the neuropsychological evaluation indicated that Andrew's problems were not attributable solely to anxiety or to an academically pressured social environment, although both most likely contribute to some extent. Indeed, it *identified legitimate cognitive issues that could become more acute within his social and instructional context*. These issues, moreover, had eluded competent school testing with reputable psychoeducational instruments. How would this profile map on to his academic skills?

Oral and Written Language

Although Andrew's spontaneous language was fairly typical, he had much more difficulty with the formal language of academics and its demands for precision, abstraction, and managing complexity. As the demands increased, his discourse would become disorganized. His scores on formal language measures were in the average range, although his word retrieval (ability to find words he needed) was less competent, only in the low-average range. Importantly, although Andrew's score on the word retrieval test could certainly be considered "normal," his obvious difficulty with finding words had the more significant downstream effect of disorganizing his language formulation, which was especially troublesome in academic situations that required him to communicate ideas with precision.

The significance of Andrew's cognitive profile for his oral and written language abilities became clear when he was asked to write. In his writing sample (Figure 8.4), Andrew described a scene from a book. Although he worked hard and included many details, his narrative is a list-like sequence of syntactically simple sentences connected by *so* and *then*, offering little context for a reader. For example, he does not explain the purpose of a soup that puts hair on one's chest. Just as he had copied the complex geometric design in a linear, incremental fashion, line by line, without distinguishing elements that were more or less conceptually important, here he lists elements of the story without weaving them into a coherent narrative or conveying motivation, essentially treating the elements of the story at face value. Furthermore, because language formulation and writing placed great demands on his cognitive resources, Andrew had trouble simultaneously attending to details such as spelling and tense, compromising the quality of his work, as his teacher had observed.

Andrew's reading was consistent. He competently read single words, and his skills were instructional, at an adequate rate, in fifth-grade-level narrative material, in which he was aided by familiar content and a strong narrative structure. Yet he read at only a frustration level in fifth-grade expository (science or social studies) material; his rate was slow, he failed to comprehend the gist, and his retelling, like his writing and his approach to the complex figure, consisted of a series of details strung together but not integrated into a cohesive thematic whole. Again, although his scores on standardized testing were competent, he faltered when asked to process lengthier, more ecologically relevant text, especially when it was not firmly anchored by familiar meaning and structure (analogous to his improved memory for the ROCF in the structured format).

This is a scene from "Jason and the
Aliens down the Street. Sudden Cooper's
invisible belt was wearing off and the
guards were able to see him. Then I
came up with a plan to rescue Cooper.
I told him the plan and Copper said
"I am a very powerful magicinen." "If
you don't let me go I will destroy you.
So you could have guessed that Lootna
and I will have to pick up things. so
Cooper decided to make me drink this
awful soup that made hair grow on your chest.
Then Cooper said "I toss Grugg the Awfuls
hat to a space in the room and it will
still be floating." So Cooper tossed the
hat into the air and I caught it. Then I
tossed it out the window and Lootna
got the crystal. Then we got out of
the fort, ~~out of~~ got in the space ship
and got ba~~th~~ck to earth.

FIGURE 8.4. Transcription, preserving line breaks, spelling, and cross-outs, of Andrew's writing sample.

Andrew's reading and writing skills, while certainly close to grade level, clearly reflect his neuropsychological profile and oral language competency. Significantly, *both are inadequate for him to compete on an independent basis within his particular educational niche.* Indeed, on state-mandated testing, his English and language arts performance barely achieved proficiency, placing him below most peers in his community.

Andrew's performance again clearly implicates *a cognitive source for his performance problems rather than anxiety or simply a competitive academic environment,* although the latter certainly complicates the effect of his functional profile. His difficulties with writing and comprehending expository text suggest a legitimate learning problem that has not been detected. Again, however, the evidence is not black and white and emerges only under certain conditions.

Mathematics

Andrew became anxious and fidgety when working with the mathematics specialist, suggesting that math triggers anxiety for him. Although he was attentive and eager to please, he was hesitant to commit himself to a response. His achievement was at the late fifth- to early sixth-grade level, with both conceptual knowledge and procedures well mastered. Although his problem-solving skills were good, he adopted his characteristic linear approach. As he became more anxious, he made numerous corrections and his approach became even more rigidly linear, adhering closely to algorithms that he had been taught. On timed tests, his imprecision escalated, revealing the impact of his slow processing speed on his performance. Although the structure of mathematics helped to organize Andrew and he had a good grasp of topics, when challenged by more complex problems, especially applications for which he did not have a ready algorithm, he would revert to his linear style and his precision would suffer, as his teacher had noted.

Andrew's essential cognitive profile was again evident, now in mathematics. Although well taught, with good mastery of requisite topics and skills, his performance could deteriorate when he was challenged with complexity or requirements for speed. His anxiety in response to math suggested that he experiences math as more challenging, perhaps because he needs to come up with one correct answer. This anxiety could further compromise his performance, leading to self-doubt, especially on tests, despite his mastery of topics. Thus, the mathematics evaluation was highly consistent, but interestingly, it was only here that Andrew's anxious tendencies began to surface, suggesting that *he experiences situationally specific anxiety, interacting with the cognitive issues.*

Psychology

Andrew did not easily express his feelings, but he could be quite expressive when he played sports, an area of clear strength, confidence, and satisfaction. He was described as empathic, expressing concerns about family members who might be sad or angry. Standardized behavioral questionnaires revealed no areas for concern, but Andrew could be vulnerable to situational anxiety, primarily related to academic performance. Thus, *Andrew's anxiety was a response to, rather than a cause of, his problems.*

Diagnosis: The Child–World Interaction

Based on school testing, competently executed with well-regarded psychoeducational instruments, Andrew fit none of the designated categorical boxes and thus could not be *identified* as having a learning disability. But there remains the long history of recurring questions about academic performance in a diligent and motivated boy, and the vague but persistent intuition, on the part of Andrew's teachers and parents, that something was not right. There were also his subpar scores on the NCLB testing, which involves more complex and ecologically relevant curriculum-based material. In the context of this contradictory picture, the evaluation provided the basis for constructing Andrew's *child–world system* and resolving these apparent contradictions. Of the four hypotheses entertained at the outset, only one survives as primary: namely, that cognitive issues, for which he has been partially able to compensate, undermine Andrew's performance. His tendency to become anxious, his excellent prosocial values, and the educationally pressured community in which he lives play key contextual roles as well.

The team concluded as follows (emphasis added):

> "Andrew is a nearly 11-year-old fifth-grader of solid cognitive potential whose profile is marked by vulnerability to complexity and a slow pace of processing and output, the effect of which may be exacerbated by anxiety and difficulty communicating his wishes and emotions. Andrew's language expression and organization problems most likely feed into his difficulty verbalizing his thoughts and feelings. Cognitively, Andrew tends to adopt a linear and deliberate approach, and does not easily see the frameworks and concepts that organize the material and make it more comprehensible. Although he often will grasp these concepts after more extended time and exposure, he does not immediately do so, and his production can thus be slow and effortful. *As he moves on to the middle school, with the increased demand for managing larger volumes of material more fluently and providing organization for his own efforts, he will need support and close monitoring in order to be able to manage the curriculum comfortably.*
>
> "In terms of his academics, Andrew's greatest areas of difficulty involve reading comprehension, especially in expository text, and writing skills. At the end of the fifth-grade year, he is only at a frustration level in expository text, and thus *will be at a growing disadvantage in terms of the reading and writing requirements of content-area subjects (e.g., science, social studies)*, as he may struggle to extract information from these texts and to express his ideas at a more abstract level. This is of *particular concern in a relatively fast-paced and competitive school system.* His mathematics skills are better established. He has been well taught, and given time, he can effectively summon and implement strategies at the late fifth- to early sixth-grade level in terms of curriculum."

Why, however, were Andrew's difficulties so invisible to a standard, well-respected, and competently administered psychoeducational test battery? How can we resolve this apparent contradiction? In striving to maximize their psychometric properties—reliability, validity, scalability—developers of many standard psychoeducational tests must use test items that are relatively discrete and do not mimic the more typical challenges faced by a child in a classroom, particularly higher-level integrative demands of the upper grade levels. Andrew could be vulnerable to complexity and he had difficulty integrating large volumes of details to make meaning, but his ability to manage more discrete elements of these tasks was intact when he was not overwhelmed by the information load. As a consequence, he was successful on these psychoeducational tests, thereby disqualifying himself from support or even recognition of his problems. Nevertheless, it was clear to his family and to his teacher that something was not up to par. The more ecologically motivated and neurodevelopmentally informed evaluation, although admittedly less psychometrically sound, clearly documented the source of his struggles.

Recommendations

Recommendations are aimed at restoring equilibrium to the system. One component was modest remedial support in specific areas of skill development. Equally or more important, however, was to provide the adults working with Andrew with a more accurate shared understanding of his profile so that they could gear expectations appropriately and implement accommodations in a manner that made sense within his particular school setting. In terms of actual resource commitment, the demand would not be great.

The specific recommendations included direct support for written language and metacognitive skills, a flexible and supportive learning environment with a relaxed pace, and a willingness on the part of content-area teachers to accommodate Andrew's difficulties with written expression and expository text. It was also recommended that he not take a foreign language at the middle school level in order to devote more time to writing skills and general strategy development, that he be placed in a moderately paced mathematics class, and that consideration be given, if needed, to professional support to help him manage his anxiety and express his needs verbally.

What Happened?

Near the end of the seventh grade, Andrew's mother reported that the evaluation had reassured her by confirming her long-standing intuition that something made learning a little more difficult for him than it should be. Talking to the teachers and having testing through the school system had not really given her answers. She had hoped that the evaluation would identify a specific learning disability and that the diagnosis would lead to some kind of "cure." Unfortunately, as is so often the case, that did not happen. Andrew's problems were not the result of a discrete defect that could be isolated and cured, but of a complex of cognitive and ecological factors. In such cases, the evaluation more frequently serves to describe and hopefully to reframe the problem, directing everyone's efforts to common and well informed approaches that are likely to be more productive.

The evaluation had been completed at the end of the fifth grade, just as Andrew was to move to middle school. The elementary school staff did not read the reports since Andrew would be in the middle school, and the middle school staff wanted to "wait and see" how he did before considering them seriously. Andrew's mother met with the guidance counselor to assure that someone had read the reports, but Andrew could not be formally identified as a student with a disability. The school testing had not documented a need for services, and Andrew was making effective progress. She was assured that the children who qualified for services had more significant needs than Andrew—which was undoubtedly true. The recommendations provided in the reports, many of which would not have necessitated direct services, and even the description of the cognitive profile, were not acknowledged in any formal way by the school nor were they read by Andrew's teachers.

Andrew's mother did manage to have him assigned to a learning center for students who needed extra help but did not qualify for services. He was also excused from music class in the sixth grade to give him more study periods because the volume of homework had become such a burden. But Andrew did not seem to get much out of the learning center, and his mother needed to monitor what went on there. With no apparent alternative, she reluctantly assumed the role of his academic support system.

With his mother's daily support, Andrew was reasonably successful in the sixth grade, achieving mostly A's and B's. But she needed to check everything he did to make sure that he understood the material. Whenever she let him work more independently, his performance would slip. On the one hand, because Andrew got so much help at home, his teachers could not appreciate his struggles; on the other, because he was so well intended and responsible, his mother could not let him experience the failure that would need to occur in order for them to do so.

A positive outcome of the evaluation was that Andrew's mother felt less frustrated with him at home. Before the evaluation, she would wonder why he was not focusing on what he was doing, and she would become frustrated when she thought he knew the material and then did not do well on a test in school. Now, with the understanding she had gained, she recognized his legitimate difficulties, and she was more inclined to be understanding than to feel angry or frustrated. Still, she felt inadequate as his support system because she was not a teacher and did not always know how to work with him.

Writing, as predicted, emerged as Andrew's biggest problem area. Since her own strengths lay more in math, his mother struggled to provide help in his area of greatest need. Moreover, her role as his academic support had become a significant burden on the family. She had two other children to care for, yet the homework had become her daily responsibility. She tried to communicate the extent of her burden to the school, but they reassured her that they did not perceive an issue.

In the seventh grade Andrew's grades were now more consistently B's. His schedule included more study periods to get some of his work done before he came home. The family had considered hiring a tutor, but that would be one more burden on his already busy schedule. Andrew played sports year round, and his athletic successes were a major boost to his self-esteem, as were his very positive social relations with his friends. His mother wisely chose not to take away from his rewarding time in those areas. He had been placed in the lowest level of math in sixth grade, which made him feel bad about himself, and he was pleased when he was inadvertently moved up to the middle level. With support from home, he had been able to hold his own in that class, which his mother felt was positive for him psychologically. Although he always got his homework in correctly and worked diligently, he did not always really absorb the material or know what questions to ask if he did not. At one point she let up a bit; he failed an important math test and blamed himself for being "dumb." Now her work with him no longer just made the differences between A's and B's, but between passing and failing.

As children become adolescents, they often assert their independence and can balk at working with a parent. Andrew generally did not complain about his homework load or working with his mother; but he did display a bit more "attitude," and there were occasional battles about homework. Still, because of his very compliant and responsible character, he generally accepted the need to work with her.

As for the future, Andrew's parents are squarely focused on surviving middle school, and they are hopeful that high school will work out better because of its greater flexibility in the choice of courses and levels. Andrew's mother maintains a healthy developmental perspective on his learning issues. She reassures Andrew that "what matters is that you find something that you like to do and that you can be good at and ... it doesn't matter that you get all A's.... Right now it seems like that's

what's important, but you'll find out later in life that that's not important." The research literature bears this out as wise advice.

Commentary: The Developmental Perspective

Like most developmental phenomena, Andrew's learning situation has
multiple layers: His neurodevelopmental profile is embedded in his temperament and values, in his family, school, community, and society. His
cognitive profile put him at risk; from early on, he showed language and
fine motor delays, and his vulnerability resurfaced each time he faced
a new academic challenge. But his problems were never severe enough
to earn formal recognition, in part because of his very compliant and
well-intended character. He clearly depended on his context for support,
flourishing with some teachers and languishing with others. Moreover,
his issues were not specific to his oral and written language abilities but
reflected his more general cognitive profile. Predictably, his risk escalated
in middle school, as his vulnerability to complexity collided with a more
demanding curriculum and without the support of a primary classroom
teacher who might or might not "get him." His profile, moreover, very
much fit that of the LI-NA, learning impaired–normal achieving, group
described in Chapter 5: His problems emerged most prominently in the
context of demands for fluent processing and production as well as integration of larger volumes of more complex or abstract information.

But there were other salient contextual issues. Had he been a more
rambunctious youngster who was easily frustrated and became an irri-
tant in school, had his mother been less willing or able to commit herself
to his educational success and to do so effectively, had his school and
community been less aggressively academic, his story could have been
quite different. Had he not derived satisfaction from his athletic and
social achievements, his self-efficacy and motivation might have been
more significantly eroded. In a variety of situational contexts, Andrew's
investment and achievement could easily have fallen further behind, and
then he might have qualified as learning disabled or come to be viewed
as a behavior problem.

Although one might be tempted to view the school as the villain
in this piece, that would be unfair. From the school's perspective, there
are indeed many students in greater need of resources. Andrew is well
behaved and continues, in their view, to do well, although his performance occasionally falters, and he causes no trouble. His scores on psychoeducational testing were exemplary. Moreover, the system is simply
not set up to deal with children such as Andrew. The primary goal of the
school testing is not to better manage Andrew's educational situation
but to make a determination as to whether he qualifies for special educa-

tion resources. In a sense, he was penalized for his diligence and good behavior as well as his mother's heroic efforts.

Although Andrew did not meet criteria for special consideration by school testing, the stress associated with his situation could have been greatly alleviated by a nonconfrontational forum, with a constructive goal of problem solving, within which the lengthy written evaluations obtained by his parents could have received an officially sanctioned reading. Such a forum would have provided teachers with a shared understanding upon which to interpret his behavior and make appropriate accommodations and modifications, as well as a basis for communication between home and school. With better communication, Andrew's mother might not have had to assume her intensive role as support system. Within the existing legal framework, however, Andrew's legitimate learning issues could not be recognized.

Equally important and easily overlooked are children's strengths and competencies. Andrew clearly has important strengths, both personal and cognitive, and he has the capacity to become a successful adolescent and adult in myriad ways. Yet school, by challenging him in his areas of greatest difficulty, is leading to a cascade of increasing frustration and self-doubt. His difficulties, albeit legitimate, are largely curriculum based, in the sense that all children are expected to achieve at the same level in the same ways, within a relatively narrow bandwidth. With more diverse options, his situation would undoubtedly be different. Ultimately, the challenge is not so much to normalize his skills in these "deficient" areas as to direct him in ways that play to his strengths so that school does not become a source of demoralization and distorted self-concept. If, however, the expectation is that students such as Andrew will participate successfully in terms of specific standards, then the dysfunction in the child–world interaction needs to be officially acknowledged and strategies developed to deal with it more effectively.

Chapter 9

Beyond a "Reading Problem"

Things get jumbled in her brain.
—SARAH'S MOTHER

Although children are typically identified for evaluation because of perceived deficits in specific academic skills, more often than not the profile is far more complex and nuanced, with direct consequences for the child–world system. This is hardly surprising for all the reasons detailed thus far about developmental disorders. The case of Sarah illustrates the complexity that is often the reality. Even for someone who has a documentable reading or math problem, there can be no easy or meaningful diagnostic boxes. This case also illustrates the exceptional efficacy of intervention when the school, family, and evaluation team can engage collegially in a spirit of problem solving, targeted to the child's individual profile and with the shared goal of promoting successful development.

THE CASE OF SARAH

History

Sarah was a 9-year-old girl who was about to enter the fourth grade. Her mother was employed as an editor at a regional newspaper and her father as a technician in the communications industry. She had an older sister who was doing well in school. The parents were amicably divorced, both playing an active role in their daughters' lives. The family lived in a low- to middle-income exurban town. The median household income was roughly $50,000; 26% of heads of household held managerial or professional jobs, and 15% had college degrees or higher. On the state-mandated testing, 58% of Sarah's peers scored in the proficient to advanced range in English/Language Arts and 51% in Mathematics. Fourteen percent of students receive free or reduced-price lunch in school. Although this was presumably not a community with great material resources, as will become apparent, the school culture was nevertheless child centered, a crucial element in Sarah's developmental course.

As is typical, it was reading that first brought Sarah to attention. In the first grade, she had more difficulty learning to read than most of her peers, but her reading was not dramatically delayed and the difficulties were chalked up to immaturity. Things did not improve in the second grade, however, and Sarah was given Title I support as well as small-group reading and writing three times a week in the classroom. Significantly, Sarah's second-grade teacher really "got" her, and she had a reasonably good year despite her troubles. The teacher focused on her strengths, in particular, her strong verbal skills, boosting her self-confidence.

School testing was completed in May of that year. Sarah demonstrated exceptionally strong verbal skills (Verbal Comprehension, 130), with only average Perceptual Reasoning (102) and lower Working Memory (91) and Processing Speed (94). Although achievement scores on the Woodcock–Johnson–III (WJ-III) were all solidly in the average range, her overall score on the Grey Oral Reading Test–4 (GORT-4) was only a 91. Since the Conners Parent and Teacher Rating Scale scores were in the clinical range for both hyperactivity and inattention, an ADHD diagnosis was entertained. Projective testing revealed anxiety about academic performance.

As a result of the school evaluation, an individualized education plan (IEP) was implemented in the third grade, with reading support provided both in the classroom and in direct instruction three times a week outside the classroom. Nonetheless, that year did not go well. The third-grade teacher did not seem as tuned in to Sarah as the second-grade teacher had been, sometimes assuming that her poor performance was intentional, most likely because of Sarah's very impressive verbal presentation. Moreover, because she could no longer compensate so well on her own, the work became more frustrating, leading to growing self-doubt. She began to falter in math as well.

At home, Sarah was displaying more stress, appearing drained when she got home after school. Changes in a child's behavior and demeanor are a primary signal of dysfunction in the child–world system. Sarah worked hard in school to make people think she was managing, but she would fall apart at home, with homework a prime trigger. In group projects Sarah would often feel self-conscious because she could not keep up, and peers would make negative comments about her difficulties. Moreover, her anxiety, which had been confined to academics, now extended to social challenges. At home she developed sleep difficulties and sought comfort in eating. Sarah was receiving counseling to deal with these issues and to support her adjustment to the divorce.

Sarah's third-grade teacher reported that all her skills were at grade level, with the exception of math and writing, which were somewhat below. The teacher perceptively noted that Sarah gives the initial impression of a confident and capable student, but that her "self-assured expressive language may mask underlying weakness." She also noted problems in oral reading fluency, in part because Sarah "does not pay attention to details," again invoking the ADHD attribution. Sarah also had difficulty spelling, consistently using conventions, and organizing ideas into a logical and complete written assignment.

As Sarah approached fourth grade, the school's plan was to modify her IEP to include in-class math support and writing support outside the classroom, in addition to her reading. Developmentally, the scope of her problems was expanding as she encountered greater contextual challenge. At this point, Sarah's parents referred her for outside evaluation because they were seeking a more definitive diagnosis than they had received from her school and wanted to find out why she had such a hard time focusing. Sarah, her mother remarked, feels that "things get jumbled in her brain." Significantly, the school was eager to use the evaluation to further adjust or refine their approaches, a positive prognostic for the child–world system. The history suggested the following hypotheses:

- Sarah's problems are referable to her reading disability.
- Sarah has an undiagnosed attention disorder.
- Sarah's academic and social problems are referable to broader cognitive compromise
- Sarah has an anxiety disorder that contributes to her problems.

Testing and Observation

Figure 9.1 illustrates schematically the findings from the evaluation.

Neurology

Sarah displayed slow automaticity in timed naming, corroborating a neurodevelopmental basis for the learning problems. Her performance was equally slow for symbolic (Letters and Numbers) and nonsymbolic (Colors and Objects) stimuli. On the ADHD questionnaires, Sarah's mother documented inattention symptoms in the clinical range, but the teacher did not endorse a clinical level of either inattention or hyper-

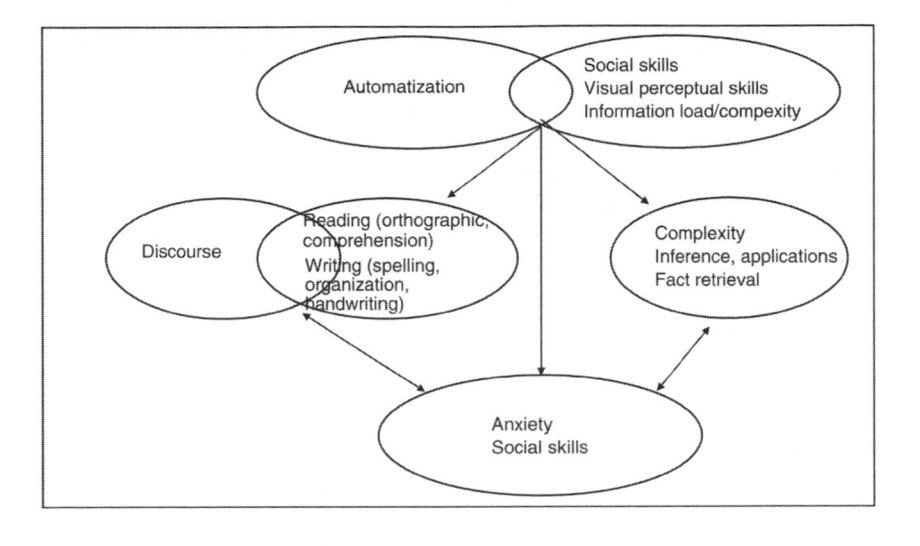

FIGURE 9.1. Schematic depiction of findings from the interdisciplinary evaluation for Sarah. Labels indicate areas of difficulty. Strengths not included here for simplicity of presentation.

activity symptoms, arguing against an ADHD diagnosis. Her strong performance on a continuous performance test further argued against such a diagnosis. The physical examination documented an increased body mass index, consistent with Sarah's mother's concerns about her inclination to eat to soothe her anxiety. In terms of the hypotheses, the neurology examination ruled out the ADHD diagnosis. The timed naming performance, moreover, suggested that Sarah's problems are not confined to symbolic material (reading) but are more broadly based.

Neuropsychology

Sarah was well invested in her performance and worked in a deliberate fashion throughout the session, with very effortful processing. Social interaction was appropriate, although Sarah's manner was intermittently reminiscent of an older or younger person. Sarah commented that things get scrambled in her brain and that she often feels that there are "too many things going on at one time."

There was, as prior testing had shown, a dramatic discrepancy between Sarah's very well-developed verbal knowledge and expression and her nonverbal and problem-solving skills, which were much less competent. She had particular difficulty with complex materials that were not anchored by meaning, especially if they were perceptually challenging. On the Rey–Osterrieth Complex Figure Test, Sarah focused on individual features without recognizing the broader context and framework (Figure 9.2). She failed to detect a meaningful pattern, distorting the design substantially. Her recall, as a consequence, was highly fragmented with significant loss of information, especially the elements of the organizing framework. As she worked, she verbally labeled each element and articulately observed that "I remember pieces." When the design was presented to her again in the structured format, her perfor-

SARAH

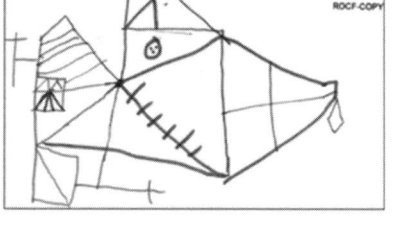

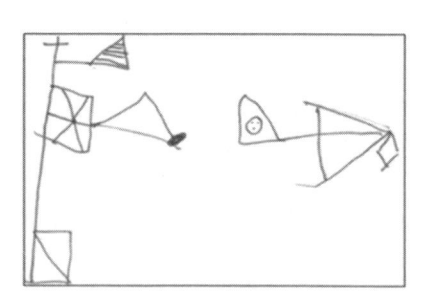

COPY   IMMEDIATE RECALL

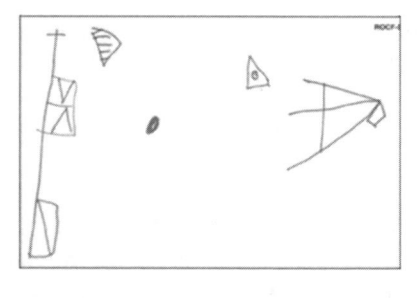

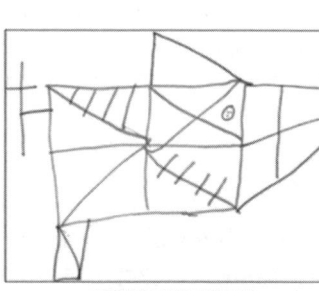

DELAYED
RECALL

STRUCTURED
PRESENTATION
IMMEDIATE RECALL

FIGURE 9.2. Rey–Osterrieth Complex Figure Copy, Immediate Recall, and Delayed Recall productions as well as Immediate Recall after structured presentation for Sarah.

mance improved substantially, indicating the extent to which she can benefit from structure and reframing.

Sarah also tended to misprocess details, especially in visually challenging materials, which a teacher could interpret as carelessness. On the Block Design subtest, she was supposed to copy geometric designs using colored blocks. Sarah was effective on the easier items, but as they became complex, she did not recognize when her productions were discrepant from the model, often significantly so. She similarly misprocessed details that were not firmly anchored in meaning, such as random digits (Digit Span) and proper names (CMS Stories), with associated distortion and confusion.

Sarah's excellent verbal knowledge and expression masked her fragile mastery of problem solving, concept development, and details, especially with visually or perceptually complex information. She was most comfortable in material anchored by concrete meaning. In visual materials, in particular, she would miss or distort details and thus make seemingly careless errors. These in fact stemmed from inefficient processing or difficulty using patterns to monitor herself. In general, she had difficulty integrating details into a meaningful and coherent whole, adopting an arduous piece-by-piece strategy, often without appreciating intent or context. Similarly in social situations, she would miss the intent of an interaction when she could not easily integrate the multiple and simultaneous verbal and contextual cues. Inferential reasoning would be particularly challenging for her; she was more comfortable when ideas were communicated explicitly. Sarah's perception that "there are too many things going on at once" stemmed from her difficulty integrating multiple cues into a meaningful context and her tendency to perceive information, whether academic and social, on a piecemeal basis. Yet her sophisticated verbal presentation gave others the impression that she could understand and solve problems at a high level—which was not necessarily the case.

In terms of hypotheses, the neuropsychological examination identified a cognitive profile that would manifest itself in multiple arenas. It corroborated Sarah's observation that things were jumbled in her head and further suggested a cognitive source for her anxiety. She would become insecure and anxious as complexity increased, despite her excellent vocabulary and sophisticated verbal presentation.

Oral and Written Language

Sarah did well on formal measures of oral language competence, and her informal conversational skill was well developed. Tellingly, however, she had more trouble using language in a more academic context, such as retelling an episode from a familiar story. Her difficulty organizing and planning language, discrepant from her excellent vocabulary, reflected her more fundamental difficulties in managing complex information.

Sarah had prominent difficulty with reading and writing, more so than her teacher had recognized. In reading, she demonstrated an early-third-grade instructional level as she entered the fourth grade. She struggled to read more complex words, sometimes perplexed by words with less common vowel patterns and two or more syllables. Her passage reading was slow and her comprehension vulnerable. Thus, although she had certainly made progress as a result of her instruction, Sarah was not yet independent at a level that would serve her comfortably in class. Because her oral language was so strong, her reading problem likely involved visual processing to a greater extent than is typical, consistent with the neuropsychological examination.

As is often the case, although the early reading problems had been addressed with some success, Sarah's underlying profile now emerged more prominently in her writing, which was significantly delayed for her placement (Figure 9.3). As her oral language performance forecast, she had difficulty generating and organizing language she planned to write. She also had handwriting difficulties, and her spelling was limited to relatively early phonetic representations. Consistent with a visual etiology, her spelling errors had a dyseidetic quality (e.g., *hete* for *heat*); she accurately applied phonetic principles to spelling, but had more difficulty generating accurate orthographic images. The multiple demands of writing were so overwhelming that the whole became less than the sum of the parts.

Mathematics

Although Sarah's skills were generally appropriate for her placement, she could be challenged by more complicated problems, such as more complex subtraction with regrouping. Moreover, her ability to apply her mathematics knowledge to real-world situations (i.e., thought problems) was only at a basic level, consistent with her difficulties with inferential reasoning and her need for structure. Sarah's efforts were further compromised by inefficient access to one-digit arithmetic facts, consistent with her poor automatization.

Sarah approached math using linear, step-by-step strategies, supported by verbal mediation, much like her execution of the Rey figure. When problems involved more than three steps or elements, she became entangled in the details and lost appreciation of overall thrust, undermining her organization. She would be vulnerable when new, more complex topics were introduced and could fail to appreciate conceptual goals

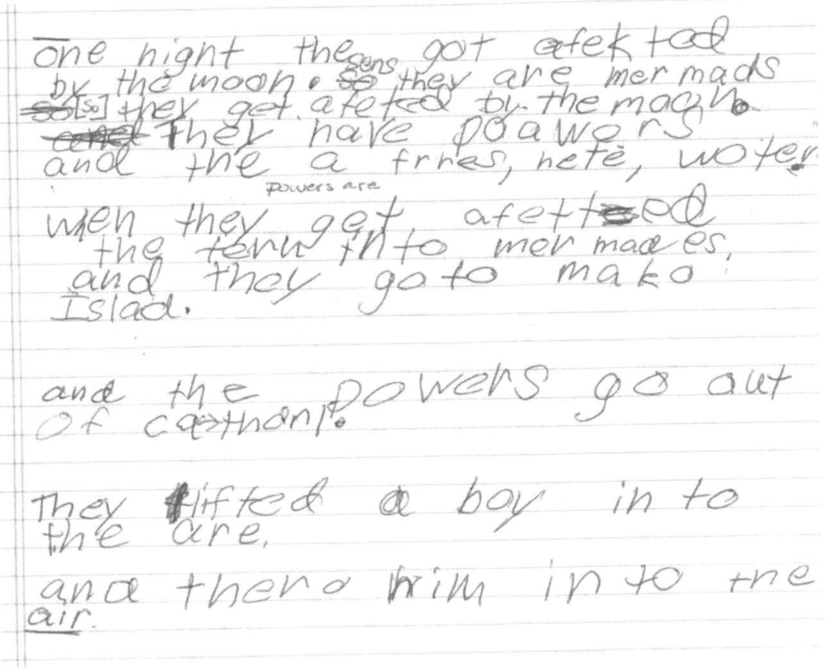
one night the gens got afektad
by the moon. so they are mermads
so [so] they get afeted by the magn.
and they have poawors
and the a frres, hete, woter
powers are
wen they get afetted
the tern into mer mades,
and they go to mako
Islad.
and the powers go out
of cathanl.
They lifted a boy in to
the are.
and thero him in to the
air.

1 /one night they got affected by the moon since they are mermaids/
3 /[so] they get affected by the moon/
4 /they have powers/
5 /and the powers are freezing heat water/
6 /when they get affected they turn into mermaids/
7 /and they go to Mako Island/
8 /and the powers go out of control/
9 /they lifted a boy into the air and throw him into the air/

FIGURE 9.3. Sarah's writing sample and corrected transcription.

while focusing on the mechanical aspects of arithmetic procedures. She could also have difficulty with longer calculation procedures that required her to merge and integrate multiple subroutines. Of particular concern as Sarah approached fourth grade was the likelihood that she would encounter difficulty applying her skills beyond basic levels. Thus, although she was managing to keep up with the late-third-grade curriculum, her cognitive profile predicted escalating risk in the fourth grade. Again to the school's credit, the math difficulty had been identified and a component added to her IEP.

Psychology

Sarah was struggling with considerable emotional distress related to her academic struggles. She was highly motivated and concerned about pleasing others. She would be at particular risk as her cognitive vulnerabilities were challenged. Not surprisingly, Sarah's self-esteem and sense of self-efficacy were fragile and vulnerable to erosion. The projective testing confirmed that Sarah's understanding of social information could be inaccurate, as predicted, largely because she could not pull all the pieces of a social situation together into a comprehensible whole. Although she had excellent prosocial values and good intuitive appreciation of emotions, Sarah and the characters in her stories had trouble asserting or executing these values.

Thus, Sarah's cognitive profile and struggles with learning contributed to, and were interrelated with, her substantial emotional distress. This distress manifested itself in internalizing problems—anxiety, withdrawal, sleep and appetite disturbance, and verbal expression of concerns. She felt supported by her family and teachers, who recognized and appreciated her strengths. These protective factors would be important for her positive development, academic and social. In terms of the hypotheses, the psychology evaluation documented anxiety, but it was secondary to her cognitive difficulties with academics and understanding and managing social situations.

Diagnosis: The Child–World Interaction

The interaction between Sarah and her world was dysfunctional in a number of respects. Although her IEP was appropriate in terms of the amount of services provided, the program was falling short because Sarah's teachers did not have an accurate appreciation of her overall profile. They did not recognize how hard she was working to try to keep pace (even though she appeared to make careless errors and to be inattentive). Nor did they appreciate the extent to which her problems were or were not under volitional control. Similarly, they did not appreciate the extent of her distress. Even though the IEP was reasonable on paper, what was missing was a comprehensive understanding of the basis for her struggles that could guide teachers in their moment-to-moment responses to her, allowing them to become better informed and thus *active participants* in her intervention. The team summarized Sarah's situation as follows (emphasis added):

> "Sarah is a delightful girl whose overall cognitive potential is difficult to characterize, with considerable strengths in verbal

knowledge and expression undermined by prominent difficulties apprehending the big picture and integrating multiple details, especially when the content is perceptually demanding or is not well anchored in familiar meaning. Sarah herself has remarked to her mother that 'things get jumbled in my brain.' Faced with such complexity and confusion, she adopts a deliberate, linear approach without appreciating the overall context or the intent of the material. Her strong verbal skills, however, can easily mask the underlying fragility of her problem solving, as her teacher observed. She also exhibits subtle compromise in aspects of social pragmatics, not appreciating nuances in interactions or demonstrating mastery of these subtle nuances in her expression. These issues, which also derive from her cognitive profile, may interfere with peer interactions as well as academics, despite her warmth and good intentions. All of this can heighten Sarah's insecurity, as she is well aware of her confusion, and this insecurity can fuel her anxious tendencies, which in turn can further impair her ability to manage the demands. Her mother reports that she maintains a confident exterior while she is at school, but "falls apart" when she gets home, indicative of the *effort she needs to invest to comply* with the demands of school and the toll that this effort may take on her psychosocially.

"Another key feature of Sarah's profile is her tendency to misprocess details, especially in visually challenging materials. This tendency has appeared to her teacher to be trouble with self-monitoring and editing. These processing errors, which are often outside of her awareness, can *give the impression that she is inattentive or perhaps unmotivated*, when in fact she is struggling to process information accurately and is very diligent and well intended. Sarah's vulnerability to misprocessing visual detail has direct consequences for her reading and writing, which have features of dyseidetic dyslexia. That is, she does not easily and automatically process the visual features of written words and does not build automatic associations between the visual representations of words and their lexical representations (i.e., word knowledge). This lack of automaticity has a direct impact on her reading fluency, as she needs to deliberately sound out words one by one rather than shifting to a more automatic and less effortful strategy of direct word recognition. Moreover, she will be vulnerable to detail errors in her reading and writing, and may not be aware that these errors have occurred. This slow and deliberate rate of processing and output is prominent throughout Sarah's work and is undoubtedly a source of stress

TABLE 9.1. Representative Test Scores from Sarah's Evaluation

WISC-IV (scaled score)		
Information	13	
Vocabulary	14	
Digit Span	11	
Coding	10	
Block Design	10	
Rey–Osterrieth Complex Figure		
Copy Organization	10%ile	
Immediate Recall Organization	< 10%ile	
Delayed Recall Organization	< 10%ile	
CMS Stories (scaled score)		
Immediate	15	
Delayed	14	
Delayed Recognition	11	
D-KEFS Color–Word Interference (scaled score)		
Color	4	
Word	3	
Interference	8	
Interference Errors	7	
	Parent	Teacher
Behavioral Rating Inventory of Executive Functions (*t*-score)		
Behavioral Regulation Index	58	57
Metacognitive Index	77	52
Wechsler Individual Achievement Test— Word Reading (standard score)	97	
Bader Reading and Language Inventory (grade 2)	Instructional early grade 3	
Analytical Reading Inventory (grade 3)		
Qualitative Reading Inventory–IV (grade 4)		
Mathematics Diagnostic and Prescriptive Inventory	Mid- to late-grade 3	
Behavior Assessment System for Children–2		
Parent	At risk: Anxiety, Somatization, Withdrawal, Attention Problems, Activities of Daily Living	
Teacher	At risk: Learning Problems, Attention Problems	

Note. WISC-IV, Wechsler Intelligence Scale for Children–IV; CMS, Children's Memory Scale; D-KEFS, Delis–Kaplan Executive Function System.

for her academically. She may also need extended time to absorb new ideas, in both her academic and social worlds, and to integrate this new knowledge with her prior knowledge and understanding.

"In terms of academic skills, Sarah's reading is instructional only at the early-third-grade level, and even at that level her rate is quite slow. The quality of her writing is also suggestive of dyseidetic dyslexia, with poor spelling and appreciation of the visual, or orthographic, aspects of words. Although Sarah's mathematics skills are appropriate for a mid- to late-third-grade student, closer to her placement, *she is likely to be at significant risk going forward because of the fragility of her problem solving and applications of formal mathematics.* She does not yet have a solid appreciation of the concepts that support mathematics algorithms. Her insecure mastery of concepts is likely to affect her ability to apply her skills independently, as her teacher has noted."

Sarah's world had both significant risk and protective elements. In school, she was approaching the fourth grade, which would greatly escalate academic demands, and thus the potential for further frustration. Social interactions, especially among girls, were becoming more complex and nuanced, and Sarah was experiencing stress in this arena as well. Yet Sarah's world also provided important protective factors. At home, she had supportive and understanding parents, who would mobilize on her behalf. Moreover, the school had been forthcoming with her IEP. Especially promising, they expressed interest in learning from the evaluation to work more effectively with her.

Recommendations

Although the recommendations are presented in list form, in fact they function systemically. For example, improving academic skills would have a direct impact on Sarah's anxiety. In addition, reframing attributions would allow the adults involved with Sarah to approach her more effectively, reducing frustration for everyone. With this understanding, everyone would be better prepared to make decisions.

1. Endorse IEP: The current IEP was endorsed, but recommendations were directed to the content of the services. For example, Sarah should focus on exposure to text rather than decoding in her reading instruction. *[Sarah is especially vulnerable in situations in which she needs to integrate details in service of a broader goal or sequence of*

steps. Thus, a focus on component skills, or individual specialist services, without attention to metacognitive strategies would limit the efficacy of intervention].

2. Modify attributions: Teachers would need to appreciate that Sarah's problems are not confined to specific academic skills but *would manifest themselves throughout the curriculum.* Direct services would need to be carefully integrated with classroom instruction, and Sarah's general education teacher should be prepared to offer consistent support and accommodations. Metacognitive skills should be developed throughout the curriculum. *[Although it seems basic, reframing attributions can be among the most important components of an intervention plan. Reframing can empower teachers to intervene more appropriately on a moment-to-moment basis. Sarah needs support throughout the curriculum, not just in specific academic skills. Moreover, children like Sarah, who have difficulty with integration and complexity, can be confused by multiple services unless they are explicitly integrated into the classroom.]*

3. Monitor anxiety: Teachers should be vigilant for escalating anxiety and intervene early to reframe a task, as needed, so that Sarah can work more confidently. She should be encouraged to advocate for herself to let teachers know when she is confused. *[Sarah is vulnerable to school-related anxiety, which signals cognitive overload. Although she will often try to hide it, teachers should be sufficiently aware to look for it and to intervene to help her meaningfully reconnect with the material.]*

4. Content subjects: Sarah should be exposed to grade-level content material with appropriate accommodations, even though her written work will not consistently meet requirements. Evaluation should not be tied to her literacy skills. *[Although Sarah has an excellent verbal knowledge base, her literacy skills lag significantly. She will be highly vulnerable to frustration and anxiety in content-area subjects that she is capable of understanding, requiring supportive adaptations to make the curriculum accessible to her.]*

5. Homework: Homework should be carefully monitored to assure that Sarah is not excessively burdened. Adjustments should be made from school, in terms of the amount and content of homework, so that Sarah can become independent and complete her work successfully. She could start her homework in school, with supervision as needed, so that she can function more independently at home. *[Sarah has been manifesting her anxiety and distress at home, often triggered by homework assignments that overwhelm her. Calling attention to the impact of this problem and establishing a good understanding between home and school*

can alleviate some of this burden, not only for Sarah but also for her very supportive family.]

6. Self-confidence: Sarah needs carefully orchestrated successes to bolster her self-confidence and increase her motivation to internalize supportive strategies, as well as to counter her growing sense of helplessness. Areas of interest and competency should be nurtured, both in and out of school, again to bolster Sarah's self-confidence and ability to engage actively in rewarding activities. *[Sarah's anxiety and discouragement directly affect her self-confidence and ability to engage academically. As her second-grade teacher understood, honoring her strengths is key to maintaining engagement and alleviating anxiety. The affective aspects of learning need to be addressed along with the cognitive. Often, there is a tendency to dwell on the deficits without adequate attention to competencies. Yet it is her interests and competencies that will, in the long run, be the basis for successful adult adaptation. These should be recognized and nurtured throughout Sarah's development, especially as she becomes adolescent.]*

7. Anxiety: In addition to the school-related interventions, continuing her psychotherapy would help her manage her anxiety. She would also benefit from a curriculum-based social skills training program to help her better appreciate social situations and learn strategies for managing them. The emphasis should be on developing problem-solving skills as well as greater assertiveness.

What Happened?

Late in the fourth-grade year, Sarah's mother reported on her progress. In terms of the evaluation, she said that they knew that there was more going on than just reading. Because Sarah was so articulate, she herself was able to express that "things didn't feel right in her brain." Echoing other parents, she would have preferred to hear that Sarah had dyslexia or another simple diagnosis with a label. Nevertheless, as a result of the evaluation, the parents had a clearer understanding about how she processes information. That understanding was validating not only for them but also for Sarah, who understood intuitively and had expressed that something was wrong. Sarah's drawing of the Rey figure was a vivid demonstration for her parents of how she processes information. They understood that she struggles to take things apart and put them together again in her mind. Even if they had no name for her diagnosis, they now understood "what it was like for her in her head."

Having that understanding helped Sarah's parents deal with her more effectively, not only when they helped her with homework, but also in day-to-day tasks. Their more informed approach has greatly decreased the tension for her in all areas of her life. They had always known that they needed to be patient with her, but they did not know how to go about it. They now understood that her problems would not be resolved, but that addressing them constructively would be a continuing process as she developed. They now aim to manage her problems rather than move past them. This has helped everyone relax and focus on easing challenges rather than attempting to "cure" her inability to deal with them. Sarah herself was eager to learn about the evaluation and excited to have her feelings validated.

As foreshadowed by their initial response to the testing, the school staff was exceptionally interested and willing to adapt the IEP to better meet her needs. Even though it was summer, the principal immediately scheduled a meeting before the reports were available, reassuring Sarah's mother of the school's commitment. Early in the fourth grade, the team reviewed the reports page by page, figuring out how to institute each recommendation. Accommodations were introduced: Someone was assigned to Sarah in class to keep her focused and on track; Sarah was given extra time for writing assignments to allay her anxiety; small-group testing was offered in some situations. Because so many children came and went in her classroom, Sarah did not feel different. Sarah's mother would remind the teacher of Sarah's needs if there was a problem, and because the teacher was receptive, things typically worked out. With their more informed understanding, teachers could be proactive in her management. In situations where Sarah feels competent, she needs no accommodations. She excels at projects and oral reports, where her exceptional verbal skills and knowledge are an asset.

In terms of her academic skills, Sarah has made impressive gains. Following the reading specialist's recommendations, the emphasis shifted from single-word decoding to increasing exposure to text, starting at a comfortable and accessible level. Sarah has now nearly caught up to her grade level; she enthusiastically reads chapter books that would have defeated her a year ago. In her mother's words, she is "soaring." Although spelling is still a struggle, as she gains more exposure to text, her spelling has improved as well. Sarah manages in math with assistance. As predicted, she can be initially overwhelmed by multistep problems, especially word problems, but with assistance she is successful.

Sarah has also made encouraging gains in her social skills and comfort level. After a few conversations with the teacher early in the year, she learned to feel comfortable expressing her need for assistance when she was overwhelmed. With the help of her social skills group, she is now far less anxious about potential social issues on the playground and less inclined to take things personally. Sarah continues to work with her therapist every few weeks and likes to use the sessions to manage her stress. The anxiety still comes and goes depending on circumstances, but is generally much decreased.

Finally, Sarah is making excellent progress controlling her weight. Rather than instituting a rigid weight control program, her parents helped her to become more sensitive to the health value of what she eats and provided opportunities for exercise. She regularly participates in swimming, yoga, and horseback riding, which she loves, and she has come down a full size in her clothing.

Commentary: The Developmental Perspective

Sarah's story stands out largely because of the very significant academic and mood problems that were present when she arrived for evaluation and the substantial gains that she made. This success is due, in no small part, to the receptive and cooperative stance of her school as well as her parents' willingness to accept results that were difficult to hear and adopt a constructive attitude toward the information. Sarah's relief at the identification of problems that were not previously recognized and her willingness to engage constructively with the support that was offered also worked to her advantage. Moreover, the portrait of the child–world system generated by the evaluation promoted a shared understanding not only of her profile, but of the particular strategies that would be needed to help Sarah adapt more effectively to the demands of school and, equally, for the school to adapt to the needs of Sarah.

Although only minimal changes were required in the structure of the IEP (i.e., commitment of resources), the shared understanding of the source of Sarah's academic problems, the impact of those problems on her stress and anxiety levels, and the social implications of her cognitive profile were all essential to improving the equilibrium of the child–world system. For example, the school's open attitude toward changing the emphasis in reading instruction, as her profile required, led to dramatic gains in her reading. Their ability and willingness to provide the social skills curriculum greatly alleviated Sarah's growing social anxiety. More than any specific curricular intervention, however, the shared goal of problem solving on Sarah's behalf was fundamental to her dramatic gains.

Chapter 10

Learning-Disabled Children Grown Up

This chapter considers the longer-term developmental trajectories for three learning-disabled children who were evaluated as part of the research program described in Chapter 5. The stories of Nora, Aaron, and Annie provide an important perspective on development and adaptation, echoing many of the research findings described in Chapter 4.

THE CASE OF NORA

She is finally living in her competency.
—NORA'S MOTHER

History

Nora was a charming 9-year-old who was just entering the fourth grade in her local public school. She had always struggled with school, and her parents and tutor were concerned about her poor progress in reading and math. Her father was a free-lance photographer and taught photography in a private school; her mother worked as an acupuncturist. Nora was an only child and had arrived in the world as a cuddly and sociable infant who would become anxious unless she was held. Her sociability and her vulnerability to anxiety would reemerge as themes throughout her development, playing off against her cognitive profile in salient ways. Nora's learning issues were not a "stand-alone" problem; their significance would be powerfully influenced by their context, both internal and external.

Even before she entered kindergarten, Nora's parents had concerns about her academic skills. From an early age, she could memorize books that were read to her, but she could not pick out letters from a page and did not pick up phonics from *Sesame Street*. The foreshadowing of her difficulties was not limited to literacy; she also had trouble with puzzles. The difficulties with puzzles hinted that Nora's cognitive troubles would not be manifest in a specific "dyslexia" and that the broader cognitive context would play a key role.

Nora entered kindergarten in the local public school. Although she did poorly on a readiness test, the teachers discounted the results because she functioned so well in class. This would be the first, but not the last, instance in which Nora's social skills would deceive teachers into missing the depth of her academic struggles. Her social gifts would prove to be both a protection and, ironically, a risk for her. Now a young adult, Nora recalled this dynamic clearly:

> "In school I was really anxious, I was really stressed out. It was hard for the teachers to see that I had a problem because I was so good in school, I never acted out."

Nora's parents continued to be concerned about her academic progress, requesting testing in the first grade. The team concluded that Nora's problems were "developmental," but they nevertheless provided an IEP that included reading support and speech–language therapy. Although she was consistently well behaved and engaging in school, she began to have tantrums at home when it came time to do homework. Her parents engaged a private tutor, who implemented a standard phonics-based reading approach. With this added support, she began to make significant progress.

By the end of the third grade, however, math was the major problem. The teacher observed that Nora had difficulty seeing and applying patterns, reminiscent of her troubles with puzzles. By the end of the third grade, her IEP included math services. Meantime, in response to her parents' continuing concerns, the school completed more testing. On an IQ test, Nora's verbal skills were above average, but her nonverbal skills were only in the average range. Her academic skills were, however, quite delayed—reading in the 25th percentile and math only at the 12th percentile.

This evolution of a learning disability profile, as we have already seen, is not unusual. As curricular demands shift, the neurocognitive profile will manifest itself in different academic areas. In Nora's case, the cognitive profile was further complicated by her intense desire to fit in with peers. Because she was so socially sensitive and aware, she was easily embarrassed by her academic troubles, and this sensitivity exacerbated their impact on her.

The Evaluation

It was at this juncture that Nora's parents brought her for the independent evaluation. Her teachers reported that her skills were somewhat below grade level in reading, writing, and spelling, but far below in mathematics. Science and social studies were adequate. Most of her in-school services at that point were now directed to math. At the same time, the teachers described her personal qualities in glowing terms:

> "Nora is delightful! She has a certain level of poise and maturity. She has wonderful verbal skills and enjoys sharing her outside experiences with the class. Nora is a hard-working student. She always does her best. She is kind, polite, and respectful. She is helpful to others or in solving conflicts."

But they did note academic concerns, writing that "She is concrete in her approach to writing and math activities." In addition to her difficulty with patterns, they noted problems with "remembering and applying previously learned information" and with "directional skills and sequencing." The teachers noted only minor concerns about anxiety on a standard questionnaire, endorsing only "overly anxious to please," "worries," and "self-conscious."

Nora presented similarly for her evaluation. She was socially delightful and exhibited no overt signals of anxiety. The neuropsychologist noted a somewhat literal cognitive style, trouble with concept development, and effortful and awkward motor output. Perhaps most significant, *she was easily overwhelmed by complexity and would then revert to linear strategies, executed in a hard-working, deliberate way, to compensate.* This theme would be echoed throughout the evaluation, most importantly in her language and academic skills. Neurologically, Nora's examination revealed mildly dyspraxic features and slow and awkward motor output, confirming a neurodevelopmental basis for her learning difficulties.

In oral and written language, Nora did well on discrete language tasks, but was more vulnerable when speed and complexity characterized the tasks, in a manner that she would encounter in a typical classroom. She again reverted to linear, step-by-step approaches to manage the load and was prone to misinterpret more complex language—which would certainly increase her burden throughout the curriculum. As she entered the fourth grade, her reading skills were instructional only at the second-grade level, well below the school's estimate. Her writing was similarly delayed, with numerous spelling errors and simple syntax, as well as poor mechanics and labored handwriting. Nora relied on her good knowledge base to comprehend spoken and written language, but this compensation strategy would not sustain her in higher grades.

Nora's math skills were, as the teacher had indicated, significantly delayed, estimated to be at the late-second to third-grade level. Place value concepts (tens, hundreds, etc.) were not yet established, and Nora had particular difficulty applying her skills to real-life situations. Again, she deployed a linear, deliberate approach, becoming obviously frustrated with writing when she tried to use paper and pencil. Consistent with the neuropsychological profile, Nora faced her greatest challenges in math when she encountered complexity—a troubling signal as she entered the fourth grade.

Psychologically, Nora was a delightful and highly motivated girl. She displayed a mature understanding of other people and their emotions, as well as leadership qualities among peers. She did, however, exhibit temper flares around homework. Nora expressed sadness and distress about her learning issues, harbingers of more acute problems to come, but these emotional concerns were restricted to academics, and she was otherwise well adjusted. In retrospect both Nora and her parents recall significant distress in elementary school. Yet at the point of the evaluation, she was not yet showing significant psychological or psychosomatic symptoms.

The evaluation certainly confirmed skill delays that exceed what school observation and testing had revealed. As she entered fourth grade, Nora struggled with late-second-grade skills in reading, writing, and math. The skill delays, however, were only one element of her profile. Her cognitive profile, it was predicted, would soon affect all academics; vulnerable to complexity, Nora compensated by mounting an effortful step-by-step approach to meet perceived demands without effectively appreciating concepts. Her oral language would become an increasing problem with more challenge. Given her profile, Nora was working very hard indeed for her accomplishments, and still falling short. Complicating the effect of her cognitive profile, of course, was her distress, which, combined with her excellent social skills, sensitivity, and her intense desire to fit in with peers, made academics an even more emotionally charged area of her development.

The impending challenge of the fourth grade and Nora's social concerns raised warning flags. The team observed in its summary that "*Nora is at particular risk this year with the increased complexity of demands.*" The team recommended expanding her IEP, not only in terms of allocation of services, but to include accommodations throughout the day, especially in metacognitive skills and adaptations to output demands.

Significantly, the team recommended that "given Nora's tenacious desire to … blend in with her peers, she will need some help in understanding and accepting the nature of her learning difficulties. Identifying a person at school who could meet with her over time and explain the issues … will be important."

That same year Nora and her family volunteered to participate in the study described in Chapter 5. Figure 10.1 displays her performance on the information-processing battery (recall that for these tasks, a *high score denotes poor performance*). Her scores placed her at high neurodevelopmental risk for academic problems, even at the basic level of information processing. Figure 10.2 summarizes Nora's performance on the more standard neuropsychological testing from the study. Her written language performance was below par and oral language above par. Most striking, however, were her poor visuospatial reasoning, processing speed, and motor function. Thus, Nora was clearly struggling with issues that put her at academic risk well beyond the confines of reading or math, and these would constitute a significant burden as she struggled to manage daily classroom demands.

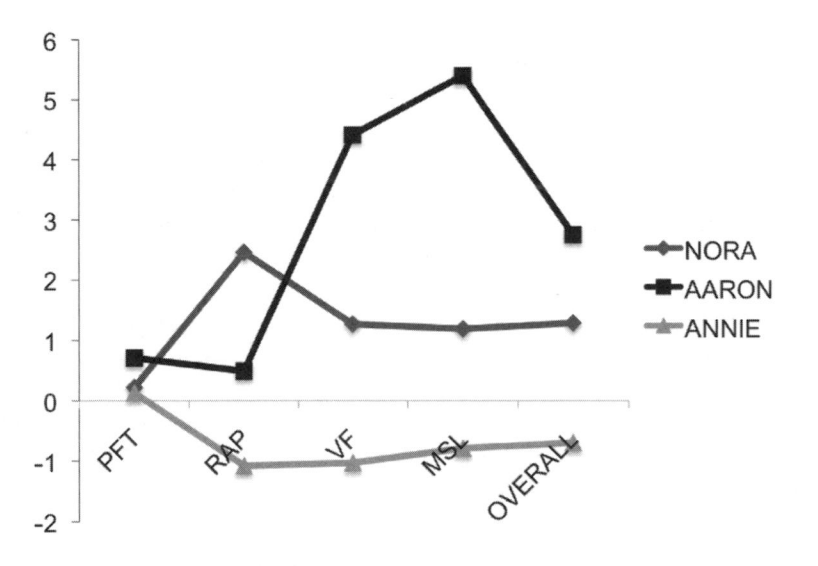

FIGURE 10.1. Performance of Nora, Aaron, and Annie on low-level information-processing (LLIP) battery described in Chapter 5. Scores are standardized to a mean of 0 and a standard deviation of 1; *higher scores indicate poorer performance*. PFT, paced finger tapping; RAP, rapid auditory processing; VF, visual filtering; MSL, motor sequence learning.

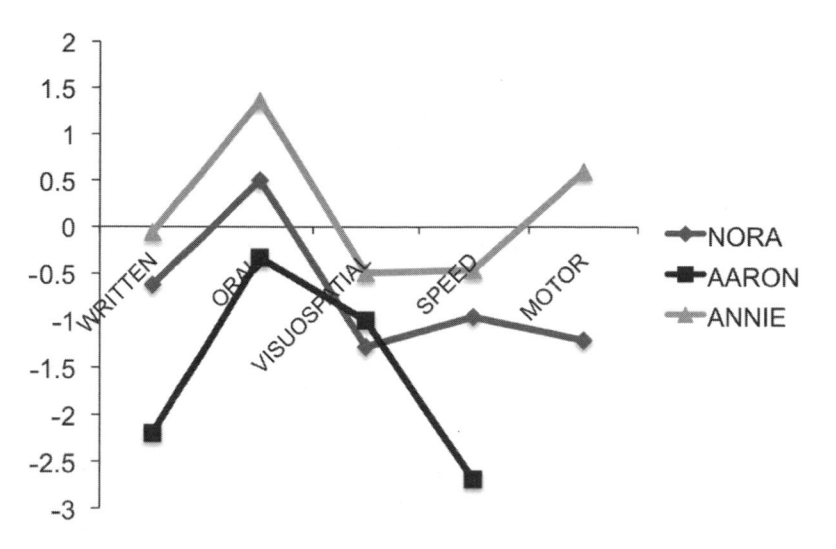

FIGURE 10.2. Factor scores from clinical neuropsychological testing for Nora, Aaron, and Annie. Scores are standardized to a mean of 0 and a standard deviation of 1; *higher scores indicate better performance.*

After the Evaluation

Nora's parents felt vindicated by the evaluation, which had documented significant cognitive, academic, and emotional issues that needed to be addressed. In retrospect, however, this vindication was "only the start of the battle." Even though she continued to struggle, the school minimized Nora's issues, saying that "she's not up to speed" or "she's still developing," and many of the recommendations were not implemented or taken seriously. The staff did not seem to comprehend the magnitude of the experience for Nora, not just academically but emotionally, in part because of her cheerful and sociable demeanor.

Nora, however, became increasingly distressed as the curricular demands escalated and, as had been predicted, she was less able to cope. She did not want to call attention to herself; despite her profound academic struggles, she was intensely determined to be just like everyone else. Nora's social skills were an asset, in that she was well liked by teachers and peers. But they were also a liability, since she conveyed a false sense of well-being and allowed teachers to minimize the depth of her distress. Meanwhile, because of her anxious temperament, her stress was being expressed through troubling physical symptoms and unhappiness that were all too apparent at home.

As the fourth grade progressed, the situation unraveled. Nora would work very hard in school and came home exhausted. Moreover, in school she would not apply the effective skills and strategies she had learned from her private tutor because she did not want to call attention to herself. Nora was by then pulled out of class for special education support for half of her instructional time and had great difficulty with this model, both academically and socially. Her academic program had become increasingly fragmented and contradictory, and she was expected to integrate what she was being taught by several special education teachers in school, the general education setting, and her private tutor. Yet as the evaluation had highlighted, Nora's skill deficits were embedded in a broader cognitive profile, a major feature of which was her great difficulty in perceiving and making connections. This fragmented model, while providing hours of support on paper, served only to further confound her. Socially, the program was adverse to her psychological makeup, magnifying her feelings of being different. For Nora, being singled out as different was tormenting and further exacerbated the already significant cognitive struggles she was having.

Nora's behaviors at home—not only her escalating distress with homework but her physical symptoms—had reached an alarming level. It was clear that something had to be done. The school's resources, for whatever reason, clearly could not and would not serve her, and her mental and physical health appeared to be in significant jeopardy. Nora's parents, in consultation with her tutor, pursued a full-time special education setting. For Nora, the school was miraculous, more from a psychosocial perspective than even an academic one. According to her mother,

> "The school rebuilt Nora's confidence. She had friends. She started to like herself, and she did not see herself as a freak.... Overall she was happier, her load was lighter."

Nora, too, speaks glowingly of her years at that school:

> "It was awesome. It's a really great school.... Within the first year you could see a huge transformation in my attitude. I was coming out of my shell. It was really great because I actually felt like I was doing well in school, and I was happy. I stopped being so anxious and nervous. I really started to learn how to advocate for my needs and use my voice, and become the person who I actually was."

The legal and financial challenges, though, were daunting. Because Nora's family did not have the financial means for the very costly tuition, they were thrust into a legal battle with the school district. Moreover, the relationship between the family and the public school had become so adversarial that it was no longer tenable for her to return there if the private option did not work out. Nora's mother withdrew her retirement savings to pay the tuition, eventually recovering a portion of the costs.

Nora made good academic progress at the new school. She learned to read and did well in her classes. The overwhelming benefit, though, was to her mental health. Her physical symptoms abated, and she was happy. Moreover, her considerable strengths outside academics were widely recognized as assets. In eighth grade Nora won the award for the student who best exemplifies the value system and program at the school, with a unanimous vote from her teachers. At graduation, she received a standing ovation—a remarkable moment for a family that had been through so much.

Unfortunately, that school did not have a high school program and, in any case, Nora's parents were simply unable to afford more tuition. She would need to go to public high school, but could not do so in their town. Ultimately, with reservations about all the schools they saw, they elected to move to a nearby town where they attended church and had a supportive community. Nora's experience was mixed at best. The school was academically oriented, with most students attending college, and Nora found it stressful. She was given special education support for organizational skills, and although she could now read, she did not enjoy it and forced herself to do the reading. She pushed herself to do things she saw others doing, and in her sophomore year enrolled in some honors classes. She made friends, but was embarrassed about going to special education, concerned that others would not respect her as a student.

As the years went on, Nora once again became increasingly stressed. Her physical symptoms resurfaced, causing numerous absences, and her grades dropped. Nora still feels that this negative turn of events was not because of her learning disability or stress, but because she was not as dedicated to school as she could have been. By the end of her senior year, she was exhibiting significant school avoidance, and she just managed to graduate. Looking back, Nora reflects that her main emphasis in high school was her friends, not her academics. Although the family's relationship with the school was not adversarial, these were difficult years. Whether Nora did not do well because she did not invest effort, or whether she did not invest effort because she could not cope with the demands and atmosphere of a competitive suburban high school remains an open question. The bottom line was that school was stressful, academics were difficult, and Nora, like most people, gravitated to her strong suit, in her case, her social skills.

Although Nora applied and was accepted to college, she and her family decided that college did not make sense for her at that point. Her mother found a postgraduate community service program that intrigued Nora. She applied, surprising her parents by requesting a placement on the other side of the country, causing some trepidation after her difficult high school experience. Although Nora worried about going so far away, this was what she really wanted to do, and her parents wisely supported her independence.

Nora was assigned to work with bilingual children in a school in a low-income immigrant neighborhood. Here, with this new beginning in a niche where her strengths and competencies were highly valued, her gifts took a front seat, and she thrived. Moreover, she was able to act independently on the positive values instilled in her by her family and her church community. She committed herself "120%," volunteering every Saturday for community service projects with the children. Significantly, the headaches that had plagued her throughout high school disappeared. She had always loved to work with children, and she resonated with the values of the program. She was given a lot of responsibility and spent much of her time tutoring second graders in reading and math. Nora recognized herself in these children, and she was troubled that so few of them would be adequately supported because the resources were so limited and the children were not well understood. She loved the hands-on nature of the work, even organizing a camp. The leadership potential and prosocial values Nora had demonstrated as a young child and at the private school once again came to the fore. Her self-confidence was restored by work with which she was genuinely engaged and could be successful.

Nora's learning issues still affect her life, but only in small ways, such as when she needs to write a check and accidentally transcribes a number wrong. She knows she needs to take her time to get things right. But she is living independently, managing her own finances, and excelling at a challenging job where she is respected and contributing in important ways to her society. Significantly, Nora finally feels that she is in an environment where people are less judgmental, and she is comfortable seeking help. "I've always been worried and embarrassed about making mistakes," she says, "but people [in the program] are not going to judge you and that's huge." As for the children, she wants not only to help them academically, but to be a positive role model for them.

In terms of the future, Nora's plans are still unformed. She plans to work in the nonprofit program for 1 more year. Eventually she will go back to school, but how or when is uncertain. As her mother so aptly puts it, she is finally able to "live in her competency," and that has been a wonderful experience for her. She has also seen that there are different ways of achieving life goals, including, but not limited to, attending college. She is enjoying her competencies rather than struggling with, and hiding, her difficulties.

Commentary: The Developmental Perspective

Nora clearly struggled with significant learning difficulties. At the level of basic information processing, her impediments were at the more severe end of the spectrum. For Nora, however, the *meaning* and thus impact of her neurobiological profile was determined in large part by developmental and contextual factors. From a developmental perspective, her social gifts and her anxious temperament declared themselves early in life and would shape her course in many ways. Whereas some children with similar cognitive profiles might have been less bothered, or might have displayed behavior problems in the classroom that would have forced more intensive intervention, Nora cared so much that she managed to disguise or minimize her problems in school. She participated in a *folie à deux* between herself and the school that allowed the school to minimize the problems while her problems festered.

By the fourth grade, as predicted, Nora's considerable adaptive strategies began to fail her. Because of her anxious nature and fierce desire to do well, the dysfunction between the "child" and the "world" began to manifest itself in internalizing physical symptoms and distress, the developmental cascade. Further adding to her considerable risk was the acrimony that had developed between her family and the school. Such discord is a known risk factor for adverse psychosocial outcomes. Whether any plan within the context of a public school environment could have worked for a girl such as Nora is, of course, debatable. In her case, the inclusion model, which can work well for many children, was simply toxic.

Along with the risks, Nora had a steadfast source of protection in her parents, who were strong advocates and made remarkable sacrifices to do whatever was possible to promote a good outcome for their daughter. Yet they eventually encountered the reality of their limitations. Had they had greater financial means, Nora might have had the option of attending a private high school, which might have been less stressful for her. For most families, there are no choices, and even advocacy can be limited, as parents may not have the knowledge or resources to pursue alternatives, or they may be intimidated by institutions.

Probably most striking in her case, and entirely in concert with the lifespan perspective, is Nora's coming into her own after she leaves the narrow confines of the educational system and enters the world of work, where she can act on her good values, and, in her mother's beautiful turn of phrase, "live in her competency." Her parents' acute understanding and the mutual recognition that school was not a good place for her shaped Nora's course at this point in her life. Like the adults in the Frostig School study, moreover, Nora reports that her learning disabilities have now receded as impediments in her life. Not only can she exercise her gifts, but she no longer experiences the judgmental environment of school, which is so constantly focused on evaluation and comparison with peers. Although Nora's next steps are unclear, the research suggests an excellent prognosis. Developmentally, those children who find a niche and show good adaptive outcomes in their 20s are likely to continue to enjoy success in terms of both work and family.

THE CASE OF AARON

> They really didn't teach me how stuff worked, like math.
> —AARON

History

Aaron was a 10-year-old fourth grader, the son of a single mother who had worked as a dental assistant to support the two of them. His father lived out of state, had a history of substance abuse, and was infrequently involved in his son's life. Aaron got off to a rocky start medically. He experienced significant fetal distress at birth and was transferred to a neonatal intensive care unit, where he spent the first 10 days of his life. Neurodevelopmentally, therefore, he was at increased risk. Because of his developmental issues, Aaron attended early intervention and a special needs preschool program, receiving services through kindergarten.

Early in his school career, concerns were raised about Aaron's attention. In kindergarten, he was diagnosed with ADHD and placed on a variety of medications. Stimulant medication was accompanied by the alarming emergence of tics, so the medication was discontinued. Aaron's mother took him for a consultation with a pediatric neurologist. Although the neurologist found no lingering effects of the drug, he did question the diagnosis, suggesting that learning issues should be investigated more thoroughly.

The school by then had also recognized Aaron's learning problems. In the first grade he received special education services for all his academics as well as speech and language, mostly within the classroom. By third grade Aaron was receiving pull-out services for reading and oral and written expression, as well as speech–language therapy in a small group. Still, his teachers expressed significant concerns about his attention; he was said to be distractible and impulsive. They were also concerned about his social development. He interacted more easily with adults than peers and needed teacher guidance for peer interactions. Peer relations would be a continuing theme in Aaron's development, interacting with his learning issues. Engaging in academics can be even more challenging for children with learning problems when their peer relations are distressed, making school an especially aversive environment.

Aaron was tested comprehensively in school in third grade. The academic scores were generally clustered at the mid-second-grade level, although the writing sample was scored at the fourth-grade level. Aaron's reading accuracy was at the third-grade level, but his rate was slow, at the early-second-grade level. His IQ was solidly in the average range, Verbal somewhat higher than Performance IQ. By fourth grade, Aaron was receiving daily special education support in reading and math. His IEP included one period a day for reading (with 10 students) and math help before school (also with 10 students).Yet his mother was concerned because school was such a troubling experience for him. She therefore sought an independent evaluation.

Although Aaron had a long-standing history of reading problems and average intelligence, by the fourth grade, when he arrived for evaluation, his teacher was reporting that he was far behind in all subjects. She described him as socially immature and unable to adequately process information. The teacher observed that he was highly distracted, unable to focus, and could not work independently. On a psychosocial questionnaire, she endorsed numerous problems with both attention and anxiety, as did his mother. Although the school clearly recognized Aaron's learning disabilities, the subtext of their remarks suggested that they believed his poor progress was due to untreated ADHD. Although Aaron's mother was convinced that his problem was not ADHD, she also saw attentional issues. Asked what problems she wanted help with, she first listed "To help him get less distracted and more focused" and "to help him to be less fearful." Aaron's mother also noted that he had a gift for putting things together, describing him as a highly intuitive thinker in practical, hands-on tasks. This profile would shape his developmental course.

Consistent with the pattern in the longitudinal studies, the adult Aaron recalled that elementary school was a particularly tough time for him:

> "For me that was my hardest time. Kindergarten wasn't too bad from what I remember, but from first grade to fourth grade was just awful.... I had no interest, plus they didn't teach me how these academics and things work. For instance, if you taught me how an algebra equation works, I could figure it out. Or a multiplication

system, I could figure it out. Either they taught it and I wasn't paying attention, or they just didn't teach me the right way."

In fact, the math curriculum the school used was highly verbal and
emphasized multiple approaches to a math problem, which would indeed
have been a poor fit for Aaron. To compound his distress, he suffered
socially. Although he was biracial, that was not an issue for him at that
stage in his life. Much more troubling was his weight. Weight is a major
source of social prejudice, and Aaron suffered because of it, not just
from peers, but from teachers:

> "The issue was when I was in gym class, they were against my
> weight I think. They would make me run more, they would make
> me work out more, that type of thing. The gym teachers would put
> me through things boot camp style, just because I was overweight.
> It was kind of abusive toward me."

Aaron's weight would continue to be an important contextual issue, as
would his anxiety and tendency toward social isolation.

The Evaluation

Aaron arrived for the evaluation in the spring of his fourth-grade year
as an engaging and cooperative boy, physically large, with height and
weight exceeding the 98th percentile. Although his teachers endorsed
attentional symptoms on structured questionnaires, their ratings did not
meet criteria for an attention disorder. Aaron's mother also reported
inattention, but more symptoms of anxiety. Thus, despite impressions,
the evidence for an attention disorder was not convincing, nor was Aaron's clinical presentation.

The neuropsychologist found Aaron's overall cognitive ability to be
solidly in the average range, but he tended to adopt a concrete, linear
approach when he encountered complexity, often failing to grasp organizing frameworks and concepts. His copy of the Rey–Osterrieth Complex Figure contained all the elements, but they were distorted, and he
could recall only a few isolated details. His processing speed was exceedingly slow. Aaron's reasoning in concrete nonverbal formats, however,
was impressive, indicating that he had significant competencies that
would not emerge easily in school. When Aaron was cognitively challenged by complexity, his attention would falter. When tasks were well
structured and he could rely on his prior knowledge, he was much more
attentive and effective. His handwriting was effortful and awkward,
consuming energy and rendering written tasks even more challenging.

Aaron's performance on various tasks of rapid automatized naming, a risk factor for learning disorders, was slow and labored, indicating that information processing and output, in general, were a drag on his academic effectiveness.

The oral and written language evaluation found competencies in discrete areas of oral language, but Aaron labored to manage complex, lengthy, or abstract discourse. He worked slowly and needed language presented slowly in order to understand it. In this setting he also appeared distractible; he gave up easily, needing prompting and coaching to persist, suggesting that his language difficulties were a source of his apparent attention problems. Reading and writing were especially challenging. Now in the middle of fourth grade, Aaron's single-word reading was only at the mid-third-grade level, and his text comprehension was at the frustration level for second-grade material. Even though school testing in the third grade documented second-grade-level skills, Aaron's functional reading was actually worse in more extended text. When queried, he could accurately recall basic facts, but he was unable to answer questions that required him to draw inferences and to derive meaning from what he had read. Even if he could decode the words in a text, Aaron struggled to make meaning, as is often the case. In his writing he had significant difficulty with topic development, even after an opportunity to rehearse orally, and the mechanics were poor.

Mathematics was not much better. Although standardized testing had indicated that Aaron's skills were only at the second- to third-grade level, he was being instructed in a fourth-grade curriculum with regular special education support. In the spring of his fourth-grade year, his skills remained delayed at the mid- to late-second-grade level. He had yet to consolidate place value concepts. Thus it is not surprising that he could not engage meaningfully in the fourth-grade curriculum. As in the other evaluations, he worked slowly and deliberately and had great difficulty as solutions became more complex or required him to incorporate a variety of details and merge subroutines. He also struggled to avoid reversing number sequences and even to simply write the numbers. Moreover, Aaron's language problems interfered; he had trouble with word problems and with retrieving terms and explaining his work.

Psychologically, Aaron was well behaved, but he showed signs of insecurity and erosion of self-efficacy. He was concerned not only about his academic difficulties, especially in mathematics, but also about peer acceptance. When Aaron was asked to tell stories in response to projective materials, his cognitive profile was evident. Solving interpersonal problems was confusing for him, and he often left them unresolved. Thus, a consistent profile emerged in his psychosocial functioning as well as academics, and this profile affected his ability to manage peer relationships. Moreover, Aaron was a target for teasing, in part because of his size, which he was at a loss to manage.

The team concluded that Aaron had significant cognitive problems involving language and the integration and managing of complexity, which were manifest across his academic and social development. The attentional issues, which did not meet criteria for an ADHD diagnosis, were most florid when Aaron became cognitively overwhelmed. Given the extent of his academic deficits, this state of feeling overwhelmed was likely to occur very frequently in school. Added to this were Aaron's anxiety and his vulnerability to social stressors.

The overall structure of Aaron's education plan was appropriate, but its implementation needed modification. Detailed recommendations were made about how to manage his learning and social issues within the context of his existing educational plan. For example, among the math recommendations were emphases on consolidation of place value and on connecting abstract numerals to a concrete context so that they "told a story." In reading, he would need significant work on phonemic awareness, decoding, and sight vocabulary, but also on comprehension. Strategies for setting a purpose for reading and to map stories were suggested to help him integrate the details and make meaning from text. Significantly, it was predicted that his struggles would increase as the curriculum became more demanding. Social skills training was suggested to help Aaron manage the social environment, potentially alleviating some of his anxiety.

During the summer after fourth grade, Aaron participated in the research study. His performance on the low-level information processing (LLIP) battery suggested high neurocognitive risk (Figure 10.1). Figure 10.2 illustrates Aaron's performance on the neuropsychological test battery. His performance is below average in most domains, with processing speed the most severely impaired, consistent with the LLIP findings. Visuospatial skills are relatively strong, indicating that his ability to reason in relation to concrete visuospatial materials is less affected than his ability to fluently process visual stimuli, such as symbolic material. This is consistent, moreover, with Aaron's mother's report of an intuitive thinker who is good at putting things together.

After the Evaluation

Although Aaron's mother found the evaluation informative, the recommendations were not incorporated into his educational plan, and she feared that he would not get the attention he needed in the public school. She was troubled by the way her son was regarded in school. She felt that no one valued his individuality, saw his strengths, or was invested in his success. She decided to try the local parochial school where he would have a fresh start and benefit from smaller classes and more attention. As a single mother, she could not afford the tuition, but Aaron's grandparents were able to help out financially for a while.

Socially, things improved for Aaron at the new school. The teachers made sure that the other students socialized with him in a positive way. As he put it, that was one of their rules. He felt the atmosphere was generally more positive, and his mother was very pleased. Nonetheless, he continued to struggle academically and began staying home from school—a new strategy for dealing with his frustration that would become a pattern. Aaron just did not like going. In addition, he often felt tired in the morning, which he now believes was related to his Type II diabetes, diagnosed when he was 14, as well as his anxiety. His mother had developed health issues, and he worried about being away from her. School in general made him anxious. The academic demands were overwhelming, and he began to feel hopeless. As he put it, "They'd give me a book with thousands of pages and wanted me to read. I couldn't read it or comprehend it."

By the middle of the sixth grade, the family could no longer afford tuition, Aaron was often absent from school, and in any event the parochial school informed them that they could not provide the special education support he needed. Because his experience in the public school had been so aversive, his mother resorted to home schooling, but it was clear that she could not educate him. So he returned to the public middle school for seventh grade, where he was enrolled in a comprehensive special education program.

Despite the findings of the independent evaluation, the school continued to insist that his problem was untreated ADHD. He was labeled as a behavior problem and placed with other students with behavior problems. Aaron recalls that in seventh grade he was put in the "Behavior Room" with students who threw things, swore, and did not care about the teachers. His story at this point sounds much like Benjamin's. According to Aaron's mother, the mislabeling had lasting effects on his self-regard. She says:

> "He was accused of different things, and it has lasted emotionally, just that little experience. To this day he feels a defamation of character when he is accused of something, like he is already labeled. He doesn't like that. He still has a sensitive issue there, which is understandable.... When I investigated on my own, I found that the teachers just did not get that he wasn't ADHD. The label stuck with him for years."

Eighth grade was much better, although Aaron's experience was still mixed. What turned him around that year was the teacher in his study support room. She herself had a history of ADHD, and Aaron was impressed that she had even failed eighth-grade English. She seemed to "get" Aaron and the other students and knew how to help him understand. Her respectful attitude was crucial for him. Even so, Aaron continued to skip school. He did not get into mischief; he simply stayed home because he did not want to go. He felt school was not doing him any good. The other students were not nice to him, and the teachers did not listen to him. He also lost his grandfather that year, the primary male figure in his life with whom he had been very close. His truancy became so bad that he had to go to court. The judge recognized that he was not a troublemaker, but told him that he simply had to go to school, which his mother now backed up more forcefully.

Aaron and his mother decided on the vocational–technical high school for the ninth grade. Despite his attendance problems, the vocational–technical school saw that he was a "good kid" and accepted him. He enjoyed the work, learned electrical skills, and particularly liked being sent out on jobs. Still, he continued to struggle with the idea of school, especially after having a taste of work. Peer issues were a continuing stressor. Many of Aaron's fellow students had behavior problems, and the atmosphere made him uncomfortable. Since so many students needed special education support, all of the classes were geared for special education, and some of them he actually felt were too easy. Still, he made progress. By tenth grade he had mastered sufficient academic skills to pass the state-mandated achievement tests. Nonetheless, his school aversion and attendance problems persisted.

Finally, in his junior year, Aaron dropped out of school, staying home and doing odd jobs. When he dropped out, his mother made him promise to get his general equivalency diploma (GED). After failing the exam, he enrolled in a GED preparation program at the local community college. In this program, where students were older and were in school by choice, with the goal of learning, the peer issues were no longer a problem. Most important, Aaron felt that he was respected, that the teachers had confidence in his abilities, and that they believed he was capable. Aaron now took an active interest in learning math, wanting to understand how algebra and geometry "worked." Once he made the positive decision to learn it, he worked hard and ultimately passed the GED test with flying colors. Now removed from the social atmosphere of high school, in a setting where people made a positive commitment to school, Aaron could mobilize himself and much better manage his learning problems.

Although he enjoyed electrical work and was very good at it, his social concerns again impacted his decisions. The people who were in the trade in his area were too "macho," involved in drinking and drugs, and he was uncomfortable with them. With his family history of substance abuse, Aaron and his mother are very sensitive to these issues, and he is determined to steer clear of them. Aaron sees himself differently, more of a "college person and a gentleman."

At 19, Aaron hopes to become a firefighter and paramedic. He has started a special program at the local community college that will support him to acquire the skills he will need to manage college courses. Once he finishes this program, he plans to take emergency medical technician (EMT) courses. He is spending his spare time doing physical training, working on his weight to better manage the diabetes. As for his social life, he has yet to find a peer group, spending much of his time on his own. He does have Internet friends and thinks that maybe he will make some friends through work. But he is confident that that area will work out in time. The important point to him now is that he has identified goals that are meaningful to him, and he has a positive attitude toward achieving those goals.

Commentary: The Developmental Perspective

Once again, this time in a boy with an exceedingly difficult history from the moment of his birth, the child–world system moves toward a better equilibrium after the child leaves the public school. For Aaron, social issues were crucial in determining his course. His troubled peer relationships, the persistent attribution of his problems to undiagnosed ADHD, and most significantly, the lack of understanding and respect from teachers doomed his academic course to failure, no matter what curricular intervention was offered, ending in his dropping out of school. School had become increasingly meaningless and socially aversive for him. Significantly, he recalled his eighth-grade year as relatively successful, in large part because of a teacher who accorded him respect and understanding. Most hopeful, now that he has been relieved of the social and academic burdens of school and as he has emerged from adolescence, he is taking a proactive stance in his life. With the respect and understanding of the teachers in the GED program, he confidently mastered the academic skills he needed. This sense of agency spread to his health as well, as he began to actively manage his weight and his diabetes, much as Sarah did, reversing the developmental cascade. Although he still struggles socially, Aaron has now taken control of his life and his future, and his prospects are bright.

THE CASE OF ANNIE

You're so afraid for them when you find that things just aren't going right.
—ANNIE'S MOTHER

History

Annie was the middle of three children of a corporate lawyer and a college-educated mother, who was at home full time while raising the children. Annie was a healthy baby whose early development was unremarkable. There were early hints, though, of problems in her language development. Word retrieval was hard for her. If she wanted someone to pass the salt, she clearly knew what she wanted and why she wanted it, but could not remember the name.

Annie was bright, starting kindergarten at only 4 years of age. Yet she struggled with the alphabet that year, despite lots of ABC books in her home. Her prereading skills were not very good. The teacher told her parents that she would probably "get it" when it became more important to her. By first grade her reading problems had become more apparent. She was enrolled in the Reading Recovery program and did well, but in the second grade without this support, she again fell behind.

The principal contacted Annie's mother and told her that he thought she might have a learning problem. Their standardized testing showed that she was indeed very bright, but her school achievement did not reflect her capability. The school wanted to figure out how to help her. This active investment by the school would be a major protective factor for her. The family also arranged for private tutoring, which would continue for a number of years.

In the third grade, as the challenge increased, Annie's problems became more prominent. By then, she had fallen somewhat below grade level in reading and language, but she was performing at grade level in math and social studies, and above grade level in science. Although Annie could complete her reading and writing assignments, she needed to spend more time than her classmates. She also had trouble with handwriting, punctuation, capitalization, and organizing her ideas. Because of these problems, she was placed on a formal IEP. School testing during the third grade year found her IQ to be in the superior range, but reading and language were only in the 35th percentile nationally, which would be even lower relative to peers in her higher socioeconomic community. Math was much stronger, at the 94th percentile.

Despite her academic problems and potential for frustration, Annie did not react negatively to her situation. Her mother believes that her parents' honesty with her from the beginning may have protected her from such feelings. They told her that she was smart but had some problems with reading and spelling and that she could do anything she wanted in life. Yet the same strategy did not work as well with a younger sister, who had a similar reading problem. Thus, Annie's temperament most likely played a significant role as well. Not only was she willing to work hard, but, in contrast to her sister, Annie was temperamentally less vulnerable to stress and anxiety.

Significantly, Annie's recollections of elementary school are not particularly vivid or negative. "I don't really remember it that much. I know that I had to go and get help during the school day with a special teacher for a little bit during each day." Emotionally, she did not feel particularly affected by her status as a special education student. "It didn't really affect me that much. I didn't like having to leave the classroom, but it didn't bother me that much because the kids never made fun of me or anything." Clearly, Annie's relatively easygoing temperament protected her from potential distress related to her academic skills, as did the positive regard and respect accorded to Annie and her family by the school.

The Evaluation

Annie was referred for evaluation early in her fourth-grade year. She was polite, pleasant, and sociable. The neuropsychological evaluation confirmed her strong cognitive ability. She was, however, surprisingly vulnerable when material was complex and highly detailed, especially verbal material. She retained the gist, but her recall of details was imprecise. Her difficulties were not limited to language, however. She copied the Rey figure in a deliberate, part-by-part fashion, and surprisingly, given her intellectual strength, she was virtually unable to remember it.

Thus, her neuropsychological profile was characterized by "vulnerability to complex novel material and specific difficulty managing and processing details, particularly in the context of challenging verbal material." The neuropsychologist also remarked that her "strengths should serve her well in compensating for her areas of weakness." Because of her imprecision and confusion of details, Annie was predicted to be the kind of student who could be vulnerable to seemingly "careless" errors, which she might not notice and self-correct. It would be important that teachers not overly penalize her for these kinds of errors, which she could easily overlook despite her good motivation and hard work.

The oral and written language evaluation confirmed the word retrieval problems that Annie's family had observed. Although her language competence was otherwise good, she had some difficulty organizing her oral discourse and writing. In terms of her reading skills, phonological analysis, thought to be the hallmark of reading problems, was strong. Similarly, her rapid naming, another documented precursor of reading problems, was entirely within normal limits. Annie's reading skills were at this point only slightly delayed for placement (at the late-grade-3 to early-grade-4 level early in her grade 4 year). She understood the grade-4 passage, but had trouble with the details, as the neuropsychological evaluation had forecast, and her problem now was her slow rate. She had difficulty with multisyllabic words, especially when reading from a word list when she could not use contextual meaning to help herself. Annie's writing was coherent and grammatical but lacked punctuation and was marked by poor spelling. Thus, the neuropsychological profile, which revealed problems with the processing of details and complex material, was evident in her reading and writing. The evaluator stressed rehearsed oral reading to build fluency. As a creative approach, he suggested reading plays, which offers a genuine pretext for rehearsal. Interestingly, theater would become a passion for Annie as she grew older.

Even though Annie's teacher reported that she was doing well in math, the evaluation indicated some skill delays, placing her at the mid-third- to early-fourth-grade level. She did well on concepts and math facts, but her procedures were less secure. Again, because she had trouble with details, her work could be imprecise, a particular problem in math. She also had trouble with organization as problems became more complex, again consistent with the profile. She was very effective at applying her skills to real-life problems, but less comfortable with more abstract mathematics—a profile that forecast later choices she would make. Thus, for Annie too, math was a bit of a stealth problem, emerging later as an issue when the early focus was on reading. Psychologically, despite the substantial gap between Annie's cognitive ability and her academic skills, she was doing very well, with good self-efficacy and self-regard.

The team concluded that Annie was a bright girl with mild academic delays. These delays were of significance, however, because of her cognitive strengths. For Annie, "just average" would be inadequate to support her knowledge, reasoning, and problem-solving skills. The math evaluation suggested, moreover, that she was the kind of student who is more comfortable in applications than in more abstract situations. Across the board, Annie was vulnerable to imprecision and becoming overloaded with details; she would become disorganized as the information load increased.

Annie did not really have skill *deficits*, but she was inefficient in using her skills. She would need not only support and accommodations, but also enrichment going forward, so that she would not become frustrated by her inefficiencies. Concerns were expressed from a developmental standpoint that she might have more problems going forward because of her difficulties managing complexity, with middle and high school being more challenging for her. Psychologically, she was doing very well; her resilient nature protected her from potential frustration and anxiety.

Annie also participated in the research study. In contrast with Nora and Aaron, her low-level information processing was quite good on both occasions, suggesting that she was at generally lower risk than the other two (Figure 10.1), consistent with the clinical findings. Her neuropsychological profile, while similar to that of the others, was at a higher level and thus her relatively lower functions, while only at the average range, were not so far off from the norm, and so she differed less conspicuously from her peers (Figure 10.2). The cognitive profiles bear out the finding described in Chapter 5, that children referred for evaluation with adequate achievement show very similar profiles to those of children with low achievement, but at a generally higher level. As the figure illustrates, Annie's profile parallels the others.

After the Evaluation

Although the evaluation provided some good strategies, Annie's parents were, like other parents, somewhat disappointed because they felt that it confirmed what they already knew rather than offering them a clear diagnosis with a name and a solution. Annie's mother wryly commented that they wanted someone to say something like "Give her vitamin E and she'll be fine."

Annie did well in school but continued to dislike reading because it was effortful and slow for her. Her mother worked hard to get her to read, sometimes reading to her from textbooks to give her access to content. On her own, it sometimes took her so long to decode the words that she would lose the meaning. She "could see the same word twelve times and still need to sound it out the thirteenth time." Her inefficient decoding was a persistent problem with multisyllabic words. Annie continued to receive special education support throughout elementary and middle school. Her special education classes, however, were scheduled during chorus or band, which she did before school, or during the silent reading period after lunch, so she never felt conspicuous.

By the end of the eighth grade, something clicked and reading was no longer hard for her. She even began to read for pleasure. At home, the stress associated with reading abated. No one really knows why this happened. Perhaps the special education and other interventions had worked; the best cure for fluency problems is extensive exposure to print. Or the adolescent transition may have been accompanied by neurodevelopmental processes that facilitated the connection between the printed and spoken word. We know that the brain continues to form connections, evidenced by increases in the volume of the white matter, into adolescence, and it is entirely possible that these maturational events, in combination with consistent exposure to text, provided the substrate for Annie to overcome difficulties that had been more prominent in the fourth grade. In any event, after eighth grade, special education supports were terminated, and Annie was given a 504 plan to provide accommodations for any residual problems.

That being said, Annie did not become an expert reader and writer. She still read slowly, and spelling continued to perplex her. She took some honors courses but needed to spend more time on the reading than her peers. She also needed math tutoring along the way. According to her mother, "The things that bothered her in high school are never going to change." Nonetheless, because she was bright and had appropriate accommodations, she did very well in high school, graduating seventh in her class.

Another key element of Annie's success may have been that she felt both respected and supported by her family:

> "My parents were really helpful. They're really academically driven in my family, so I had pressure to do well. But they also helped me to do well … and they made sure that if I couldn't do it, I didn't feel like a failure."

Equally, if not more, important, Annie's teachers continued to support and respect her. Her mother visited the school annually to check in with the guidance department and teachers and review Annie's profile with them. Teachers were receptive and people advocated for her in school. The guidance department communicated reliably with the teachers. Everyone honored Annie's intelligence and wanted her to succeed. According to Annie:

> "All of my teachers were really helpful. I never had any who didn't understand or try to help me. I would talk to them at the beginning of every year and my guidance counselor would talk to them."

This positive regard, as well as Annie's own temperament, most likely protected her from the potential adversities of learning issues that had plagued Nora and Aaron.

Annie is now in college. She chooses courses carefully, making sure that the reading load is not too heavy any semester. Even so, it takes her longer than many of her peers to get her work done. Although she was an excellent student in high school and her family is very academically minded, Annie did not choose a highly competitive academic route, which would have demanded intensive reading and writing or abstract math. She chose a school that would allow her to pursue a major in theater management. She knew that she would never have a career on the stage, but she loved theater and she also knew that math was a strength, so she chose a program where she could combine her love of theater with business skills. Interestingly, in the fourth-grade evaluation, she was said to be stronger in applications than in more abstract math, and in choosing business, she found a niche for that strength. She is using her considerable competencies in a more applied setting, where academic skills will not be central to her success, and she has chosen a career path in which she has a genuine and passionate interest.

Commentary: The Developmental Perspective

Annie's story is illustrative in a variety of ways. First, as is typical, her problems were most florid in elementary school and abated thereafter, but she still needed support and continues to seek accommodations. Second, her profile is typical of our adequate achievers; she shows the efficiency/integration deficits, but at a higher level. This profile might not have brought her to attention in a less competitive environment. Third, in addition to her supportive family, which all of the children had, Annie was blessed with caring and respect from school personnel throughout her career, perhaps because she was thought to be bright. The relationship between school and home was always collaborative and respectful. Fourth, Annie's resilient temperament protected her from anxiety that others in her situation might have experienced. Finally, once she left the confines of the public school curriculum, Annie skillfully defined goals for herself that would engage her strengths and not overly stress her areas of weakness, in an area of genuine interest. Annie brought the child–world system into equilibrium.

Chapter 11

A Developmental Strategy for Resolving the Dilemma

We have met the enemy and they are us.
—POGO

The goal of this book has not been to refute or devalue any of the work in the learning disabilities field; substantial progress has been made and is incontrovertibly important, as are the gains from advocacy. Rather, its goal has been to build upon this work by advancing an integrative model for understanding children with learning problems phenomenologically. In an integrative developmental model, all of the pieces assume their rightful place. The developmental framework provides perspective on the meaning of existing research and practice, its strengths, and also its limitations. This perspective can potentially stimulate a variety of actors—psychologists, neuropsychologists, teachers, parents, administrators, researchers—to think in novel and perhaps creative ways about the children with whom they work, liberated from "should" and focused more on "how." Importantly, this will necessitate a *shift from a focus on identification to a focus on problem solving*.

LESSONS FROM REAL CHILDREN

The case studies presented in this book reveal recurring themes that are surprisingly consistent. They show the impact of the learning disabilities dilemma on real children and their families. They show the systemic nature of developmental phenomena and the importance of a lifespan perspective. They show the essential contribution of neurocognitive processes that are not captured by a focus on specific academic skills or even standard and well-regarded psychoeducational tests.

Among the young people described in this book, *the single factor that best predicted a positive developmental course in school was a collaborative attitude of problem solving among the school staff, the parents, the evaluators, and the child.* In instances where this collaboration did not occur, the negative developmental cascade continued to progress, with adverse effects spreading to a wider swath of developmental functioning. Equally important was a shared attitude of respect. Every young adult who was interviewed used the word *respect*, as did the twins' parents. Sarah's case (Chapter 9) best illustrates the progress that can be made with an attitude of mutual respect and a shared focus on the best interests of the child. The principal in Sarah's school set the tone by immediately meeting with the parent, reassuring her that they were on her side, and by creating within the school a culture of problem solving and openness. Ironically, the solution did not necessarily require allocation of more resources to Sarah (although more services were called for, in some areas), but often entailed modifying attributions and using the same resources more effectively. The school's welcoming and respectful attitude toward the independent evaluation and its willingness to institute recommendations, as well as her parents' changed perspective, resulted in major gains in all aspects of Sarah's development, reversing the developmental cascade and moving her closer to a positive developmental trajectory.

Unfortunately, the current system for learning disability identification and service provision is not structured to foster such an attitude. In fact, it is hamstrung by legal requirements that can create an adversarial atmosphere, consuming resources in the struggle rather than in the best interests of the child. Although these legal requirements were well intended, meant to protect the various constituencies and guarantee rights, too often they create more problems than they resolve. Indeed, when good things happen for children, it often seems to be *despite* the system rather than because of it.

The educational and psychological literature provides an abundance of excellent strategies for teaching children with learning problems. Cognitive neuroscience is providing an ever-expanding understanding of the neural bases of reading, language, and mathematics skills. That is not the challenge. Absent a shared attitude of problem solving and mutual respect among the parent, child, and school staff, all these research efforts are of limited utility, no matter how well founded the evidence base and no matter how elegant the neuroscience that informs them. As Pogo wisely observed, "We have met the enemy and they are us."

Achieving an appropriate collaborative attitude while preserving rights will be a major challenge for the learning disabilities field as it moves forward, but it is one that must be met if the learning disabilities dilemma is to be resolved.

The Systemic Nature of Developmental Phenomena

Another consistent theme to emerge from these case studies is that, in no case, did a child have "just" a reading problem (i.e., dyslexia) or any other discrete problem. Moreover, their dynamic and interacting cognitive and affective issues were not simply "noise" in the system, but had a material effect on the child's functioning and adaptation to contextual demands. The often diffuse nature of the problem was a source of frustration for many parents, who would have preferred a clear-cut diagnosis with proven "treatment." Indeed, in every case, the evaluation discovered heterogeneous problems that affected adaptation, including in the academic skill area, that may have brought the child to attention. Even Annie, whose problems seemed most discrete, exhibited word retrieval problems and was virtually unable to recall the Rey–Osterrieth Complex Figure. Moreover, her phonemic awareness and rapid automatized naming—the typical hallmarks of a reading problem—were within normal limits.

These stories clearly illustrated the risk for a developmental cascade, as was outlined in theoretical terms in Chapter 3, when the scope of the problems is not adequately addressed. For children such as Benjamin (Chapter 7), Nora (Chapter 10), and Aaron (Chapter 10), whose learning and developmental needs were inadequately addressed, the scope of the problems expanded to become manifest more diffusely, leading to far more serious adaptive dysfunction. As these children became increasingly distressed and hopeless, they developed significant externalizing or internalizing behaviors. Nora developed headaches and other somatic complaints leading to great family distress and school absences. Aaron and Benjamin were ultimately consigned to the "behavior problems" check box, with Aaron ultimately dropping out of school. Failure to appreciate the systemic nature of these developmental processes can lead to erroneous attributions that can materially affect children's lives, often in very negative ways. Sarah, on the other hand, who was in significant distress when she presented for evaluation, showed dramatic improvement, not only academically but also in terms of her psychological adjustment, once her learning needs, both cognitive and social, were effectively acknowledged, understood, and addressed.

Commentators have often invoked the "blind man and the elephant" story to capture the state of the research literature on learning disabilities; measure any cognitive or social function, and children identified with learning disabilities as a group will be deficient. Because of the systemic nature of developmental phenomena and the very heterogeneous expression of school troubles, it is not surprising that group data can become meaningless. The resulting frustration has led to a retreat from the broader perspective, with researchers choosing to focus narrowly on specific academic skills, which are easier to target both conceptually and methodologically. Although this research is certainly important, it can be difficult to translate clinically in relation to any particular child, for whom the individual presentation can be key. Again, as Sarah so beautifully illustrates, building a model of the individual child, including the multiple cognitive and affective manifestations of child–world dysfunction that brought the child to attention, can be essential for meaningful and effective progress to occur.

The systemic nature of the problem is not limited to the child. Often, when the child–world system is significantly dysfunctional and the school response is inadequate, parents reluctantly assume the role of special educators. This dynamic was prominently illustrated for a number of these children. Indeed, Aaron's mother became so desperate she tried to home-school him at one point. When a child is at risk of significant school failure and the needs are, for whatever reason, not acknowledged or met in school, parents are caught between the proverbial rock and a hard place. On the one hand, if they do not intervene at home to help the child succeed at school, they risk a significant and emotionally traumatic experience of failure for the child. On the other hand, if they do intervene, the school may never fully recognize the depth of the child's struggles. The necessity for a parent's involvement can have major systemic implications for the family as a whole, not just the parent and the child, as the child's homework becomes the focus of family life and frustrated parents have to deal with emotional "meltdowns" that children manage to contain when at school. Significant parental involvement is thus a key marker of legitimate dysfunction in the child–world system.

Another systemic consideration is the socioeconomic milieu. Alexander and Benjamin's parents felt acutely that their advocacy was dismissed because they did not have the educational background to command respect. Their school system, meanwhile, appeared to be resource poor, and seemed to have little to offer the boys even if they were identified. These issues, in myriad ways, can significantly impede meaningful and effective progress.

The Lifespan Perspective

Learning disability is a developmental disorder. As was discussed previously, early biases in the developing system can become elaborated into a more florid profile depending, in part, on experiences and environmental challenges. The twins in Chapter 7, Alexander and Benjamin, entered the world with different levels of risk, apparently related to their prenatal development, and these different levels played themselves out developmentally, becoming much more prominent in Benjamin's functioning. Andrew, in Chapter 8, showed a pattern of subtle problems that never quite reached the level of a "disorder" on formal testing. Nevertheless, the problems were evident quite early in his life in his language and motor development, which were somewhat delayed but not enough to qualify for early intervention, and there was consistent uncertainty throughout his school career. In Chapter 10, Nora's social skills and sensitivity as well as her difficulty appreciating patterns were also evident early, as were her incipient problems with oral and written language. In a developmental model, these early systemic biases can evolve to become manifest as more pronounced effects. At the same time, experience can modify the trajectory. Aaron, for example, received early intervention for his developmental delays. His profile, although certainly significant, might have been even more severe had he not had that experience. Sarah arrived for evaluation in the midst of a developmental cascade that could have led to a very poor psychosocial outcome but was subsequently contained and redirected by excellent collaboration between home and school and a shared attitude of problem solving.

Even more profound, in terms of our understanding of the learning disability phenomena, are the longer-term outcomes, which clearly bear out the research described in Chapter 4. As young adults, Nora, Aaron, and Annie were each in the process of defining a niche where they could rely on their strengths and interests. Consistent with the research, two out of the three described elementary school as the most stressful time for them, and they fared better as they were able to find environmental contexts in which their stress points were less relevant. Nora and Aaron, in particular, achieved dramatic gains once they left the public school system. Too often, we focus intently on deficits without an equal emphasis on strengths, competencies, interests, and especially longer-term adaptation. Successful adaptation is not only about acquiring a discrete set of skills to meet societally determined standards. It is also about identifying competencies as well as niches within which these competencies will be valued. Developmental timing is also relevant. Aaron, for example, dropped out of high school. Yet when he returned to school, in a socially tolerable setting and with goals that were now meaningful to him personally, he was able to confidently acquire skills that had eluded him for years. Perhaps it was his maturity and life experience; perhaps it was the setting. In either event, his positive attitude and his mother's persistent support and faith in him led him to proactively seek out opportunities to develop academic skills, but this time on his own terms—and, importantly, with respect.

Should the field aim for a uniform standards-referenced outcome? Or should it aim for outcomes that lead to productive, satisfying adult lives, outcomes that play to competencies and strengths and support relative weaknesses? It is human nature to prefer activities that are rewarding to those that are unrewarding. High-quality skill instruction, although certainly essential to any positive outcome, is obviously inadequate to address this key issue, which becomes increasingly salient as children become adolescent.

Neurocognitive Processes: Processing Efficiency and Integration

As described in Chapter 5, the children in the research sample were quite heterogeneous in their cognitive presentations, but consistent themes were present. Children referred for learning problems were characterized by inefficient information processing and difficulty integrating more complex material to derive meaning. Three of the four children whose evaluations were presented in detail—Benjamin, Andrew, and Sarah (Figures 7.1, 8.1, and 9.1)—displayed prominent problems with automatization as well as with complexity and information load. In general, these children needed to work harder for their accomplishments than did their peers. Their efforts were often slow and labored, as reflected, for example, in their handwriting fluency or their retrieval of words or facts. They easily became overwhelmed because they had insufficient cognitive resources to deploy to the more complex aspects of tasks.

As Jansma and colleagues (2001) wrote, "The shift from controlled to automatic processing is essential in order to free up resources needed for more complex tasks" (p. 730). It is not surprising, therefore, that this inefficiency goes hand in hand with vulnerability to information load. Over and over again, the evaluations described children who became overwhelmed by more complex information and reverted to an effortful linear, incremental approach, or whose achievement deteriorated when they needed to manage multistep problems or tasks. Writing was especially difficult because of the multiple component demands that need to be orchestrated. This dynamic was clearly reflected in the academic evaluations *but was manifested differently in each child*—again, not surprising in a developmental phenomenon.

Although the term *integration* is admittedly vague and unsatisfying, it captures better than any other word available to us the nature of the challenge that many of these children exhibit when they need to derive meaning from complex information or orchestrate component operations in the service of a conceptually driven goal. Managing these inefficiencies in fluency and integration presents the greatest unmet challenge to intervention. These more domain-general processes, too often regarded by researchers as "noise" in the system, in fact merit explicit attention on their own merit.

Perhaps significantly, cognitive neuroscience research suggests that *integration* is the intimate partner of *executive functioning*. In Chapter 6 we saw that individuals who were less effective at recruiting the posterior integrative regions compensated by engaging the anterior executive regions. This recruitment of executive resources is manifested phenomenologically as greater conscious effort—an effort that consumes resources that are then unavailable for higher-level cognitive functioning. Greater involvement of these prefrontal executive regions may be manifested in more arduous and inefficient processing. This effortful and inefficient processing and production are entirely consistent with the clinical presentation of many children referred for learning problems. The source of the problem, thus, may not be the executive functioning itself but rather the underlying confusion regarding the material to be acted upon. Inefficient or ineffective integration and understanding can undermine executive functioning at a behavioral level. Similarly, the research indicates that failure to effectively "trim" or streamline neural networks is manifested in less efficient or automatic functioning. Approaches that target executive functioning as a top-down discrete skill will most likely fall short unless they acknowledge the potential significance of these dynamics.

Finally, the evaluations repeatedly illustrated that psychometrically valid tests provide *data, not answers*. Often, careful observation of the way in which the child achieved the score is more relevant than the score itself. Equally important, accurate evaluation of academic skills necessitates observation of the child engaged in tasks that are representative of actual academic demands, referenced to the curriculum. These tasks are often too complex to be included in psychoeducational tests that strive for high reliability. Andrew, described in Chapter 8, is a clear example. Although he achieved excellent scores on psychoeducational testing, precluding him from services, the interdisciplinary evaluation identified and forecast his areas of functional distress based on his responses to more typical academic challenges and an appreciation of his particular academic context. As it turned out, these difficulties emerged more prominently with each year of middle school, again cascading to involve more and more participation by his mother to keep him afloat. This legitimate distress, so clear to his family, was invisible to psychometric testing, and this invisibility deprived him not only of potential services but, more importantly, of recognition by his teachers of his legitimate problems. Such recognition could have been beneficial clinically even without a program of direct services.

LOOKING FORWARD

Once learning disabilities are appropriately situated in the context of developmental science, as a developmental problem, it becomes apparent why capturing their essence within the prevalent modular framework has been so incredibly elusive. This disorder, like many developmental problems, is not a discrete entity but a collection of diverse phenomena that are bound together by a common characteristic: the disorder emerges when normally occurring heterogeneity in children's cognitive functioning is incompatible with socially and culturally determined demands and expectations. The source of this heterogeneity is neither exclusively biological nor exclusively experiential. Rather, it is the product of coactive biological and experiential processes that propel development and co-construct these functional systems. Moreover, their meaning is almost entirely a function of societal forces.

It follows that there will be never be a bright line or a test to distinguish those who have the disorder from those who do not and thus rescue us from the identification wars. The decision about where to draw the line is ultimately a social, economic, and political one, not a scientific one. Moreover, it follows that the universe of children and adults who potentially have the disorder will share important features but will, in the end, be infinitely diverse. There will, of course, be basic principles that obtain across individuals because of the structure of knowledge and of developing cognitive systems. But in the end, each person will differ from every other one in ways that are potentially of great clinical significance, as the case studies illustrate.

From a Skill Focus to a Child Focus

The developmental approach advocated in this book shifts the focus of analysis from the skill to the child. The neuroscientific and clinical studies provide substantial evidence that skill deficits rarely occur in isolation, in the context of an otherwise perfectly functioning system. More frequently these skill deficits are part of a broader pattern of *inefficiencies in information processing* that directly affect children's abilities to function in the contexts in which they find themselves, academically and very often socially. Moreover, the profile will evolve over developmental time, presenting itself differently in different developmental epochs and with different challenges, with the risk of adverse developmental cascades if not managed effectively.

Over the years, these processing inefficiencies have been recognized, but only to the extent that they co-occur with the well-accepted modularly conceived diagnostic categories such as dyslexia and ADHD. With such recognition, the characterizations of these diagnoses have simply expanded to include them. Hence the dyslexia diagnosis, which theoretically is a specific reading deficit in the context of otherwise normal cognition, has now expanded to include problems with working memory, processing speed, automatization, and motor skills, to name a few, and similarly for ADHD. In fact, children with information-processing inefficiencies may or may not have cognitive elements that evolve developmentally to the level of a dyslexia or ADHD syndrome.

As our case studies so vividly illustrate, the whole child needs to be appreciated in order to address the adaptive disequilibrium and facilitate progress. Efforts limited to remediating an isolated skill by a particular reading program, evidence based though it may be, will often fall well short of doing so. Scores on discrete psychoeducational tests, moreover, can fail to detect problems that emerge in more ecologically relevant situations, with significant clinical ramifications. Evidence-based assessments and interventions for specific academic skills remain essential tools, but only if situated within a broader developmental framework, despite their persuasive internal logic.

After the Learning Disability Era

It follows from the developmental perspective that the learning disability diagnosis cannot, and thus will never, be clear-cut; it is inseparable from the substantial contextual meaning that we attach to it. *Learning disability* is inevitably a social construction. In the first several decades of its existence, Kirk's (1962) inspired terminology served an incredibly important advocacy role by conferring legitimacy on the difficulties of children with learning problems, helping their families gain access to the resources they needed to cope with the world they inhabited. Over time, however, it has become apparent that the rubric is inadequate to the phenomena. With the success of advocacy and increased awareness, more and more families have come forth to demand resources, most often for valid reasons. In response, the atmosphere has shifted from one of compassion and support to conflict and turbulence, as schools attempt to cope with rising demand, much of which is most likely legitimate, given the ever-escalating goals of contemporary American schooling. The goals of parents and the goals of schools, perhaps inevitably, have often diverged in ways that cause great friction and, unfortunately, work against the best interests of the child. This was regrettably true for a number of the young people in this book.

The research community, seeking to provide clarification through empirical study, eventually encountered a similar dilemma. As they submitted the prevalent understanding of specific learning disability to closer analysis, they hit the same roadblock, and skirmishing broke out in that quarter as well. Slowly but surely, they have abandoned the term *learning disability* and retreated to safer terrain, focusing on discrete skills such as reading, writing, and mathematics. The term *learning disability* has gradually receded from the scientific literature, to be replaced by *reading disability*, *math disability*, and the like.

The struggles and controversies of the past several decades are in direct proportion to the ambiguities of the landscape. The recent introduction of the response-to-intervention (RTI) approach in the federal law may well signal the beginning of the end of the learning disability construct as we know it, as does the growing popularity of the term *learning difference* as a label to replace *learning disability*. The impending demise of this terminology is of understandable concern to some advocates, who have effectively rallied around the disability model to make significant legal gains for children. It is essential that this necessary evolution not compromise parents' standing to advocate for their children's rights to a "free and appropriate public education." Yet at the same time, the need for advocacy should not stand in the way of a clearheaded appraisal of the facts as they are, not as we might wish them to be.

The Promise of Contemporary Neuroscience

As more is known about the human brain and its functional development, the core concept of dynamic distributed neural systems has become increasingly dominant, as illustrated in Chapter 6. The clinical presentation of children referred for learning problems entails inefficiencies in basic information processing and problems managing information load, in addition to various combinations of problems involving more specific cognitive processes and academic skills. It is reasonable to look for their etiology to the developmental construction of these networks. The term *network inefficiency* may not be as catchy as *learning disability*, but it may well be a more accurate descriptor of the phenomenology. Although the research base is limited, especially with regard to children with learning impairments, the network concept may provide a conceptual bridge to the future. Watching a child with learning problems try to read or write a composition, or even sign his or her name, one cannot help but be struck by the conscious effort required to do a thing that peers accomplish fluently. The network concept, as illustrated in Chapter 6, and the important link to the automatic–effortful distinction in cognitive psychology, helps make sense of this prevalent and functionally relevant feature. Slow reading, however, is often only one manifestation of a much broader cognitive profile.

Special Education and Problem-Solving RTI

In 2000, Arthur Levine, then dean of the Columbia University Teachers College, wrote an Op-Ed column in the *New York Times*. Noting the alarm about growing numbers of children being identified with learning disabilities, he cited critics who complained that the label was being too broadly applied, at great cost to taxpayers. Levine, however, saw the phenomenon differently:

> What we are witnessing is not a fad which will pass or whose excesses will be corrected. We are witnessing the start of a revolution that will transform American education forever. It is part of a revolution we are undergoing in every other aspect of American life.
>
> The United States is shifting from an industrial society to an information society. Among other things, this means there is less emphasis on mass production and more customization of products and services. (p. 33A)

Levine observed trenchantly that

> our school system was created for an industrial society and resembles an assembly line. Students are educated by age, in batches of 25 to 30. They study for common periods of time, and after completing a specified number of courses, they are awarded diplomas. It is a notion of education dictated by seat time. Teaching is the activity that occurs during the time when students are in their chairs. (p. 33A)

What many view as an alarming growth in the inappropriate identification of children with learning disabilities, Levine views as the bellwether of a potentially fundamental transition in American education, in which education necessarily moves toward increasing individualization. The current learning disability model, he argues, should eventually become the predominant model for educating *all* students; teachers will no longer function as "talking heads" but as "experts on learning styles." Moreover, he predicts that "eventually, the nomenclature will change, and we will recognize so-called disabilities for what they really are—differences in how people learn.

Rather than call them learning disabilities, we will call them learning differences."

Levine's (2000) vision is obviously compatible with the developmental orientation. The beginnings of this shift may be contained in the RTI language included in the 2005 IDEA and the enthusiasm that has surrounded it. Although the standard protocol models, which are modularly oriented and rigidly defined, are unlikely to fulfill this vision, they may well prove to be very useful within niches, such as the acquisition of early reading or math skills, for which they have largely been developed.

More promising from our perspective is the potential of the problem-solving model of RTI. Problem-solving RTI has a number of appealing features: It is sufficiently flexible to allow for a variety of approaches; it brings together teachers, psychologists, and other school personnel, along with parents, to consult and develop solutions for a struggling student; and it is open to a consideration of the multiple factors that might contribute to the student's problems. Most important, however, is the message inherent in its name—*problem solving.* A problem-solving orientation promises to shift the focus of effort and resources from identification of a learning disability to solving the student's problem—arguably the correct goal of the exercise. This orientation heralds the possibility of a profound shift in the way that we regard struggling students, perhaps even directing us toward Levine's vision. Such an approach could defuse the potentially poisonous adversarial relationships that too often develop between parents and schools, whose effects can be so damaging.

For the model to fulfill its promise, however, several prerequisites will need to be in place. First, a problem-solving RTI approach will require a *theoretical model that can flexibly integrate the multiple considerations that are important in any child's development, and that can support a process of informed hypothesis testing.* A developmental approach to learning, as outlined in this book, is likely to be much more effective than one that is based on a modular view of discrete skills, which is rooted in the industrial approach, as characterized by Levine. Prevalent strategies of curriculum-based measurement (CBM), many consisting of 2-minute tests, have minimal prescriptive value for children struggling with the complex challenges of modern schooling. They will also be insensitive for some children, potentially leading to conflict. Judgments that a child is struggling, whether based on parent or teacher report, should be respected and allowed to override what may well be a false-negative result. A parent recently recounted how a first-grade teacher told her that her child was having trouble learning to read, but then told her that the boy could not join a reading support group because he passed the test. Nonetheless, since it was plain to everyone that the boy was struggling, he was eventually admitted to the group.

Second, teachers will need *appropriate tools and expertise, with far greater emphasis on mastery of child development in teacher training*, to solve these problems. They should then be empowered and supported to act in ways that facilitate development. Teachers should not be relegated to roles of technician or bookkeeper, delivering a scripted curriculum and keeping detailed statistical records of progress based on 2-minute tests, but should become *professional developmental specialists*, from the elementary to the high school level.

More broadly, schools need to consider *what children need to learn* to become successful adults, and whether it makes sense that every student master the same body of knowledge or skills in the same way. Children are practical creatures who, like everyone else, yearn to feel successful, respected, and useful. A child who labors to craft a five-page report on the Civil War may be far more successful learning to write about a familiar topic that engages his or her own experience or interest, and maybe even more successful in a real-world curriculum (e.g., computer science, business). Of course, knowing about the Civil War is important, but the five-page Civil War essay may not be for everyone. Harking back to Dewey, the role of vocational education merits reexamination. Aaron, for example, who struggled mightily in school, much more easily mastered the academic skills that had previously defeated him as he matured and especially when he understood their real-world relevance to a goal that was meaningful to him. No less important was his need for respect. Children such as Aaron or Benjamin can often come to be labeled as *behavior problems* as the child–world system cascades into increasingly dysfunctional directions, with the unfortunate risk of lasting adverse effects.

Finally, throughout this discussion, the elephant in the room is the economic implications. Who is responsible for shouldering the financial consequences of managing these children: the education system, the medical system, parents? If we abandon the "disability" construct, who owns the problem? Will a different approach require more resources, or only redeployment of currently available resources? This pragmatic consideration, already the source of nearly unbearable stress in the system, needs to be part and parcel of any retooling. Whatever the solution may be, however, it needs to be guided by a conceptual understanding that best reflects the actual phenomena rather than tailoring our depiction of the phenomena to suit an administrative structure. Moreover, it is critical that any new economic approach *reward collaborative problem solving* rather than instigating conflict, as is currently the case.

We stand at a crossroads. Choosing a new direction will demand open minds, constructive attitudes, and creative problem solving. Although we may seek answers from science, science can only inform. Social, cultural, economic, and political forces, and especially values, will ultimately determine the pathway going forward.

Appendix

Publications of the Children's Hospital Boston Learning Disabilities Research Center

Duffy, F. H., McAnulty, G. B., & Waber, D. P. (1999). Auditory evoked responses to single tones and closely spaced tone pairs in children grouped by reading or matrices abilities. *Clinical Electroencephalography, 30*(3), 84–93.

Duffy, F. H., Valencia, I., McAnulty, G. B., & Waber, D. P. (2001). Auditory evoked response data reduction by PCA: Development of variables sensitive to reading disability. *Clinical Electroencephalography, 32*(3), 168–178.

Kirkwood, M. W., Weiler, M. D., Bernstein, J. H., Forbes, P. W., & Waber, D. P. (2001). Sources of poor performance on the Rey–Osterrieth Complex Figure Test among children with learning difficulties: A dynamic assessment approach. *Clinical Neuropsychologist, 15*(3), 345–356.

Morgan, A. E., Singer-Harris, N., Bernstein, J. H., & Waber, D. P. (2000). Characteristics of children referred for evaluation of school difficulties who have adequate academic achievement scores. *Journal of Learning Disabilities, 33*(5), 489–500.

Peters, J. M., Waber, D. P., McAnulty, G. B., & Duffy, F. H. (2003). Event-related correlations in learning impaired children during a hybrid go/no-go choice reaction visual–motor task. *Clinical Electroencephalography, 34*, 99–109.

Rivkin, M. J., Vajapeyam, S., Hutton, C., Weiler, M. L., Hall, E. K., Wolraich, D. A., et al. (2003). A functional magnetic resonance imaging study of paced finger tapping in children. *Pediatric Neurology, 28*(2), 89–95.

Singer-Harris, N., Forbes, P., Weiler, M. D., Bellinger, D., & Waber, D. P. (2001). Children with adequate academic achievement scores referred for evaluation of school difficulties: Information processing deficiencies. *Developmental Neuropsychology, 20*(3), 593–603.

Sorenson, L. G., Forbes, P. W., Bernstein, J. H., Weiler, M. D., Mitchell, W. M., & Waber, D. P. (2003). Psychosocial adjustment over a two-year period in children referred for learning problems: Risk, resilience, and adaptation. *Learning Disabilities Research and Practice, 18*(1), 10–24.

Valencia, I., McAnulty, G. B., Waber, D. P., & Duffy, F. H. (2001). Auditory evoked responses to similar words with phonemic difference: Comparison between children with good and poor reading scores. *Clinical Electroencephalography, 32*(3), 160–167.

Waber, D. P. (2001). Aberrations in timing in children with impaired reading: Cause, effect or correlate? In M. Wolf (Ed.), *Dyslexia, fluency, and the brain* (pp. 103–125). Timonium, MD: York Press.

Waber, D. P., Forbes, P. W., Wolff, P. H., & Weiler, M. D. (2004). Neurodevelopmental characteristics of children with learning impairments classified according to the double-deficit hypothesis. *Journal of Learning Disabilities, 37*(5), 451–461.

Waber, D. P., Marcus, D. J., Forbes, P. W., Bellinger, D. C., Weiler, M. D., Sorensen, L. G., et al. (2003). Motor sequence learning and reading ability: Is poor reading associated with sequencing deficits? *Journal of Experimental Child Psychology, 84*(4), 338–354.

Waber, D. P., Weiler, M. D., Bellinger, D. C., Marcus, D. J., Forbes, P. W., Wypij, D., et al. (2000). Diminished motor timing control in children referred for diagnosis of learning problems. *Developmental Neuropsychology, 17*(2), 181–197.

Waber, D. P., Weiler, M. D., Forbes, P. W., Bernstein, J. H., Bellinger, D. C., & Rappaport, L. (2003). Neurobehavioral factors associated with referral for learning problems in a community sample: Evidence for an adaptational model for learning disorders. *Journal of Learning Disabilities, 36*(5), 467–483.

Waber, D. P., Weiler, M. D., Wolff, P. H., Bellinger, D., Marcus, D. J., Ariel, R., et al. (2001). Processing of rapid auditory stimuli in school-age children referred for evaluation of learning disorders. *Child Development, 72*(1), 37–49.

Waber, D. P., Wolff, P. H., Forbes, P. W., & Weiler, M. D. (2000). Rapid automatized naming in children referred for evaluation of heterogeneous learning problems: How specific are naming speed deficits to reading disability? *Child Neuropsychology, 6*(4), 251–261.

Weiler, M. D., Bellinger, D., Marmor, J., Rancier, S., & Waber, D. (1999). Mother and teacher reports of ADHD symptoms: DSM-IV questionnaire data. *Journal of the American Academy of Child and Adolescent Psychiatry, 38*(9), 1139–1147.

Weiler, M. D., Bellinger, D., Simmons, E., Rappaport, L., Urion, D. K., Mitchell, W., et al. (2000). Reliability and validity of a DSM-IV based ADHD screener. *Child Neuropsychology, 6*(1), 3–23.

Weiler, M. D., Bernstein, J. H., Bellinger, D. C., & Waber, D. P. (2000a). Information processing deficits in children with attention-deficit/hyperactivity disorder, inattentive type, and children with reading disability. *Journal of Learning Disabilities, 35*(5), 448–461.

Weiler, M. D., Bernstein, J. H., Bellinger, D. C., & Waber, D. P. (2000b). Processing speed in children with attention-deficit/hyperactivity disorder, inattentive type. *Child Neuropsychology, 6*(3), 218–234.

Weiler, M. D., Forbes, P., Kirkwood, M., & Waber, D. (2003). The developmental course of processing speed in children with and without learning disabilities. *Journal of Experimental Child Psychology, 85*(2), 178–194.

Weiler, M. D., Harris, N. S., Marcus, D. J., Bellinger, D., Kosslyn, S. M., & Waber, D. P. (2000). Speed of information processing in children referred for learning problems: Performance on a visual filtering test. *Journal of Learning Disabilities, 33*(6), 538–550.

References

Abosi, O. (2007). Educating children with learning disabilities in Africa. *Learning Disabilities Research and Practice, 22*(3), 196–201.

Agnew, J. A., Dorn, C., & Eden, G. F. (2004). Effect of intensive training on auditory processing and reading skills. *Brain And Language, 88*(1), 21–25.

Benasich, A. A., Choudhury, N., Friedman, J. T., Realpe-Bonilla, T., Chojnowska, C., & Gou, Z. (2006). The infant as a prelinguistic model for language learning impairments: Predicting from event-related potentials to behavior. *Neuropsychologia, 44*(3), 396–411.

Bernstein, J. H., & Waber, D. P. (1990). Developmental neuropsychological assessment: The systemic approach. In A. A. Boulton, G. O. Baker, & M. Hiscock (Eds.), *Neuromethods: Vol. 17. Neuropsychology* (pp. 311–372). New York: Humana Press.

Bernstein, J. H., & Waber, D. P. (1996). *Developmental scoring system for the Rey–Osterrieth Complex Figure.* Odessa, FL: Psychological Assessment Resources.

Bocian, K. M., Beebe, M. E., MacMillan, D. L., & Gresham, F. M. (1999). Competing paradigms in learning disabilities classification by schools and the variations in the meaning of discrepant achievement. *Learning Disabilities Research and Practice, 14*(1), 1–14.

Bronfenbrenner, U., Morris, P. A., Damon, W., & Lerner, R. M. (1998). The ecology of developmental processes. In W. Damon & R. M. Lerner (Eds.), *Handbook of child psychology: Vol. 1. Theoretical models of human development* (5th ed., pp. 993–1028). Hoboken, NJ: Wiley.

Bruck, M. (1985). The adult functioning of children with specific learning disabilities: A follow-up study. *Advances in Applied Developmental Psychology, 1*, 91–129.

Buchel, C., Coull, J. T., & Friston, K. J. (1999). The predictive value of changes in effective connectivity for human learning. *Science, 283*(5407), 1538.

Burbridge, T. J., Wang, Y., Volz, A. J., Peschansky, V. J., Lisann, L., Galaburda, A. M., et al. (2008). Postnatal analysis of the effect of embryonic knockdown and overexpression of candidate dyslexia susceptibility gene homolog *Dcdc2* in the rat. *Neuroscience, 152*(3), 723–733.

Busk, J., & Galbraith, G. (1975). EEG correlates of visual–motor practice in man. *Electroencephalography and Clinical Neurophysiology, 38,* 415–422.

Campos, J. J., Anderson, D. I., Barbu-Roth, M. A., Hubbard, E. M., Hertenstein, M. J., & Witherington, D. (2000). Travel broadens the mind. *Infancy, 1*(2), 149–219.

Caplow, T., Bahr, H. M., Modell, J., & Chadwick, B. A. (1996). *Recent social trends in the United States 1960–1990.* Montreal: McGill-Queens University Press.

Carlson, R., Sullivan, M., & Schneider, W. (1989). Practice and working memory effects in building procedural skill. *Journal of Experimental Psychology: Learning, Memory, and Cognition, 15,* 517–526.

Caspi, A., Sugden, K., Moffitt, T. E., Taylor, A., Craig, I. W., Harrington, H., et al. (2003). Influence of life stress on depression: Moderation by a polymorphism in the *5-HTT* gene. *Science, 301,* 386–389.

Champoux, M., Bennett, A., Shannon, C., Highley, J. D., Lesch, K. P., & Suomi, S. J. (2002). Serotonin transporter gene polymorphism, differential early rearing, and behavior in rhesus monkey neonates. *Molecular Psychiatry, 7*(10), 1058.

Christensen, C. (1992). Discrepancy definitions of reading disability: Has the quest let us astray? *Reading Research Quarterly, 27,* 276–278.

Clifford, S., Young, R., & Williamson, P. (2007). Assessing the early characteristics of autistic disorder using video analysis. *Journal of Autism and Developmental Disorders, 37*(2), 301–313.

Cohen, M. (1997). *Children's Memory Scale.* New York: Pearson.

Collier, D. A., Stober, G., Li, T., Heils, A., Catalano, M., Di Bella, D., et al. (1996). A novel functional polymorphism within the promoter of the serotonin transporter gene: Possible role in susceptibility to affective disorders. *Molecular Psychiatry, 1*(6), 453–460.

Crawford, S. G. (2007). Specific learning disability and attention-deficit hyperactivity disorder: Under-recognized in India. *Indian Journal of Medical Science, 61*(12), 637–638.

de Kovel, C. G., Franke, B., Hol, F. A., Lebrec, J. J., Maassen, B., Brunner, H., et al. (2008). Confirmation of dyslexia susceptibility loci on chromosomes 1p and 2p, but not 6p in a Dutch sib-pair collection. *American Journal of Medical Genetics. Part B, Neuropsychiatric Genetics, 147*(3), 294–300.

DeFries, J. C., Fulker, D. W., & LaBuda, M. C. (1987). Evidence for a genetic aetiology in reading disability of twins. *Nature, 329,* 537–539.

Delis, D., Kaplan, E., & Kramer, J. (2001). *Delis–Kaplan executive function system.* New York: Psychological Corporation.

Denckla, M. B., & Rudel, R. G. (1976). Rapid automatized naming (R.A.N.): Dyslexia differentiated from other learning disabilities. *Neuropsychologia, 14,* 471–479.

de Vries, P. J., & Watson, P. (2008). Attention deficits in tuberous sclerosis complex (TSC): Rethinking the pathways to the endstate. *Journal of Intellectual Disability Research, 52*(4), 348–357.

Doris, J. (1987). Learning disabilities. In S. J. Ceci (Ed.), *Handbook of cognitive, social, and neuropsychological aspects of learning disabilities* (Vol. 1, pp. 3–54). Hillsdale, NJ: Erlbaum.

Durston, S., Davidson, M. C., Tottenham, N., Galvan, A., Spicer, J., Fossella, J. A., et al. (2006). A shift from diffuse to focal cortical activity with development. *Developmental Science, 9*(1), 1–8.

Eliez, S., Rumsey, J. M., Giedd, J. N., Schmitt, J. E., Patwardhan, A. J., & Reiss, A. L. (2000). Morphological alteration of temporal lobe gray matter in dyslexia: an MRI study. *Journal of Child Psychology and Psychiatry, and Allied Disciplines, 41*(5), 637–644.

Elman, J. (1996). *Rethinking innateness: A connectionist perspective on development.* Cambridge, MA: MIT Press.

Fair, D. A., Cohen, A. L., Power, J. D., Dosenbach, N. U., Church, J. A., Miezin, F. M., et al. (2009). Functional brain networks develop from a "local to distributed" organization. *PloS Computational Biology, 5*(5), e1000381.

Fair, D. A., Dosenbach, N. U., Church, J. A., Cohen, A. L., Brahmbhatt, S., Miezin, F. M., et al. (2007). Development of distinct control networks through segregation and integration. *Proceedings of the National Academy of Sciences of the United States of America, 104*(33), 13507–13512.

Fisher, S. E., & Francks, C. (2006). Genes, cognition, and dyslexia: Learning to read the genome. *Trends in Cognitive Sciences, 10*(6), 250–257.

Flesch, R. (1955). *Why Johnny can't read.* New York: Wiley.

Fletcher, J. M., Francis, D. J., Morris, R. D., & Lyon, G. R. (2005). Evidence-based assessment of learning disabilities in children and adolescents. *Journal of Clinical Child and Adolescent Psychology, 34*(3), 506–522.

Fletcher, J. M., Shaywitz, S. E., Shankweiler, D. P., Katz, L., Liberman, I. Y., Stuebing, K. K., et al. (1994). Cognitive profiles of reading disability: Comparisons of discrepancy and low achievement definitions. *Journal of Educational Psychology, 86*(1), 6–23.

Francis, D. J., Fletcher, J. M., Stuebing, K. K., Lyon, G. R., Shaywitz, B. A., & Shaywitz, S. E. (2005). Psychometric approaches to the identification of LD: IQ and achievement scores are not sufficient. *Journal of Learning Disabilities, 38*(2), 98–108.

Fuchs, L. S., & Fuchs, D. (2006). A framework for building capacity for responsiveness to intervention. *School Psychology Review, 35*(4), 621–626.

Gaab, N., Gabrieli, J. D. E., Deutsch, G. K., Tallal, P., & Temple, E. (2007). Neural correlates of rapid auditory processing are disrupted in children with developmental dyslexia and ameliorated with training: An fMRI study. *Restorative Neurology and Neuroscience, 25*(3–4), 295–310.

Galaburda, A. M. (2002). Anatomy of the temporal processing deficit in developmental dyslexia. In E. Witruk, A. D. Friederici, & T. Lachman (Eds.), *Basic functions of language, reading and reading disability* (pp. 241–250). Norwell, MA: Kluwer Academic.

Garmezy, N., Garmezy, N., & Rutter, M. (1983). Stressors of childhood. In N.

Garmezy & M. Rutter (Eds.), *Stress, coping, and development in children* (pp. 43–84). Baltimore: Johns Hopkins University Press.

Georgiewa, P., Rzanny, R., Gaser, C., Gerhard, U. J., Vieweg, U., Freesmeyer, D., et al. (2002). Phonological processing in dyslexic children: A study combining functional imaging and event related potentials. *Neuroscience Letters, 318*(1), 5–8.

Gevins, A. S., Bressler, S. L., Cutillo, B. A., Illes, J., Miller, J. C., Stern, J., et al. (1990). Effects of prolonged mental work on functional brain topography. *Electroencephalography and Clinical Neurophysiology, 76*(4), 339–350.

Goldberg, R. J., Higgins, E. L., Raskind, M. H., & Herman, K. L. (2003). Predictors of success in individuals with learning disabilities: A qualitative analysis of a 20-year longitudinal study. *Learning Disabilities Research and Practice, 18*(4), 222–236.

Goldstein, M. H., King, A. P., & West, M. J. (2003). Social interaction shapes babbling: Testing parallels between birdsong and speech. *Proceedings of the National Academy of Sciences of the United States of America, 100*(13), 8030–8035.

Gottlieb, G. (1992). *Individual development and evolution: The genesis of novel behavior.* New York: Oxford University Press.

Gottlieb, G., & Halpern, C. T. (2002). A relational view of causality in normal and abnormal development. *Development and Psychopathology, 14*(3), 421–435.

Gottlieb, G., & Lickliter, R. (2004). The various roles of animal models in understanding human development. *Social Development, 13*(2), 311–325.

Gresham, F. M., MacMillan, D. L., & Bocian, K. M. (1998). Agreement between school study team decisions and authoritative definitions in classification of students at-risk for mild disabilities. *School Psychology Quarterly, 13*(3), 181–191.

Grigorenko, E. L., Wood, F. B., Meyer, M. S., Hart, L. A., Speed, W. C., Shuster, A., et al. (1997). Susceptibility loci for distinct components of developmental dyslexia on chromosomes 6 and 15. *American Journal of Human Genetics, 60*(1), 27–39.

Guttorm, T. K., Leppannen, P. H. T., Poikkeus, A.-M., Eklund, K. M., Lyytinen, P., & Lyytinen, H. (2005). Brain event-related potentials (ERPs) measured at birth predict later language development in children with and without familial risk for dyslexia. *Cortex, 41*(3), 291–303.

Hallahan, D. P., & Mock, D. R. (2003). A brief history of the field of learning disabilities. In H. Swanson, K. Harris, & S. Graham (Eds.), *Handbook of learning disabilities* (pp. 16–29). New York: Guilford Press.

Harlaar, N., Dale, P. S., & Plomin, R. (2007). Reading exposure: A (largely) environmental risk factor with environmentally-mediated effects on reading performance in the primary school years. *Journal of Child Psychology and Psychiatry, and Allied Disciplines, 48*(12), 1192–1199.

Harold, D., Paracchini, S., Scerri, T., Dennis, M., Cope, N., Hill, G., et al. (2006). Further evidence that the *KIAA0319* gene confers susceptibility to developmental dyslexia. *Molecular Psychiatry, 11*(12), 1085.

Hart, B., & Risley, T. R. (1995). *Meaningful differences in the everyday experience of young American children.* Baltimore: Brookes.

Hart, B., & Risley, T. R. (2003). The early catastrophe: The 30 million word gap. *American Educator, 27*(1), 4–9.

Hasher, L., & Zacks, R. T. (1979). Automatic and effortful processes in memory. *Journal of Experimental Psychology: General, 108*(3), 356–388.

Hinshelwood, J. (1917). *Congenital word blindness.* Chicago: Medical Book.

Ho, H. Z., & Decker, S. N. (1988). Cognitive resemblance in reading-disabled twins. *Developmental Medicine and Child Neurology, 30*(1), 99–107.

Hollingshead, A. B. (1975). *Two-Factor Index of Social Positions.* Unpublished manuscript, Yale University.

Horwitz, B., Rumsey, J. M., & Donohue, B. C. (1998). Functional connectivity of the angular gyrus in normal reading and dyslexia. *Proceedings of the National Academy of Sciences of the United States of America, 95*(15), 8939–8944.

Jansma, J. M., Ramsey, N. F., Slagter, H. A., & Kahn, R. S. (2001). Functional anatomical correlates of controlled and automatic processing. *Journal of Cognitive Neuroscience, 13*(6), 730–743.

Jarvis, E. D., Scharff, C., Grossman, M. R., Ramos, J. A., & Nottebohm, F. (1998). For whom the bird sings: Context-dependent gene expression. *Neuron, 21*(4), 775–788.

Johnson, M. H. (2000). Functional brain development in infants: Elements of an interactive specialization framework. *Child Development, 71*(1), 75–81.

Johnson, M. H. (2001). Functional brain development in humans. *Nature Reviews Neuroscience, 2*(7), 475–483.

Johnson, M. H. (2003). Development of human brain functions. *Biological Psychiatry, 54*(12), 1312–1316.

Johnson, M. H., Griffin, R., Csibra, G., Halit, H., Farroni, T., De Haan, M., et al. (2005). The emergence of the social brain network: Evidence from typical and atypical development. *Development and Psychopathology, 17*(3), 509–619.

Johnson, M. H., & Munakata, Y. (2005). Processes of change in brain and cognitive development. *Trends in Cognitive Sciences, 9*(3), 152–158.

Jung, D. Y. (2007). South Korean perspective on learning disabilities. *Learning Disabilities Research and Practice, 22*(3), 183–188.

Kail, R., Weinert, F. E., & Schneider, W. (1995). Processing speed, memory, and cognition. In F. E. Weinert & W. Schneider (Eds.), *Memory performance and competencies: Issues in growth and development.* (pp. 71–88). Hillsdale, NJ: Erlbaum.

Karande, S., Satam, N., Kulkarni, M., Sholapurwala, R., Chitre, A., & Shah, N. (2007). Clinical and psychoeducational profile of children with specific learning disability and co-occurring attention deficit hyperactivity disorder. *Indian Journal of Medical Science, 61*(12), 640–647.

Karmiloff-Smith, A. (1998). Development itself is the key to understanding developmental disorders. *Trends in Cognitive Sciences, 2*(10), 389–398.

Kavale, K. A., & Forness, S. R. (2003). Learning disability as a discipline. In

H. L. Swanson, K. R. Harris, & S. Graham (Eds.), *Handbook of learning disabilities* (pp. 76–93). New York: Guilford Press.

Kavale, K. A., & Reese, J. H. (1992). The character of learning disabilities: An Iowa profile. *Learning Disability Quarterly, 15*(2), 74–94.

Keogh, B. K., & Weisner, T. (1993). An ecocultural perspective on risk and protective factors in children's development: Implications for learning disabilities. *Learning Disabilities Research and Practice, 8*(1), 3–10.

Kirk, S. E. (1963). Behavioral diagnosis and remediation of learning disabilities. *Proceedings of the Annual Meeting of the Conference on Exploration into the Problems of the Perceptually Handicapped Child, 1*, 3–7.

Kirkwood, M. W., Weiler, M. D., Bernstein, J., Forbes, P. W., & Waber, D. P. (2001). Sources of poor performance on the Rey–Osterrieth Complex Figure Test among children with learning difficulties: A dynamic assessment approach. *Clinical Neuropsychologist, 15*(3), 345–356.

Klingberg, T., Hedehus, M., Temple, E., Salz, T., Gabrieli, J. D., Moseley, M. E., et al. (2000). Microstructure of temporo-parietal white matter as a basis for reading ability: Evidence from diffusion tensor magnetic resonance imaging. *Neuron, 25*(2), 493–500.

Lareau, A. (2003). *Unequal childhoods: Class, race, and family life*. Berkeley: University of California Press.

Leppanen, P. H. T., Richardson, U., Pihko, E., Eklund, K. M., Guttorm, T. K., Aro, M., et al. (2002). Brain responses to changes in speech sound durations differ between infants with and without familial risk for dyslexia. *Developmental Neuropsychology, 22*(1), 407–422.

Levine, A. (2000, December 22). Tomorrow's education made to measure. *New York Times*, p. 33A.

Liu, W.-C., Gardner, T. J., & Nottebohm, F. (2004). Juvenile zebra finches can use multiple strategies to learn the same song. *Proceedings of the National Academy of Sciences of the United States of America, 101*(52), 18177–18182.

Luciano, M., Lind, P. A., Duffy, D. L., Castles, A., Wright, M. J., Montgomery, G. W., et al. (2007). A haplotype spanning *KIAA0319* and *TTRAP* is associated with normal variation in reading and spelling ability. *Biological Psychiatry, 62*(7), 811–817.

Luria, A. (1973). *The working brain: An introduction to neuropsychology*. New York: Basic Books.

Luthar, S. S., & Latendresse, S. J. (2005). Comparable "risks" at the socioeconomic status extremes: Preadolescents' perceptions of parenting. *Development and Psychopathology, 17*(1), 207–230.

Lyytinen, H., Ahonen, T., Eklund, K., Guttorm, T., Kulju, P., Laakso, M. L., et al. (2004). Early development of children at familial risk for dyslexia—follow-up from birth to school age. *Dyslexia, 10*(3), 146–178.

Lyytinen, H., Ahonen, T., Eklund, K., Guttorm, T. K., Laakso, M.-L., Leinonen, S., et al. (2001). Developmental pathways of children with and without familial risk for dyslexia during the first years of life. *Developmental Neuropsychology, 20*(2), 535–554.

MacMillan, D. L., Gresham, F. M., & Bocian, K. M. (1998). Discrepancy between definitions of learning disabilities and school practices: An empirical investigation. *Journal of Learning Disabilities, 31*(4), 314–326.

Marston, D., Muyskens, P., Lau, M., & Canter, A. (2003). Problem-solving model for decision making with high-incidence disabilities: The Minneapolis experience. *Learning Disabilities Research and Practice, 18*(3), 187–200.

Masten, A. S., Roisman, G. I., Long, J. D., Burt, K. B., Obradovic, J., Riley, J. R., et al. (2005). Developmental cascades: Linking academic achievement and externalizing and internalizing symptoms over 20 years. *Developmental Psychology, 41*(5), 733–746.

Mastropieri, M. A., & Scruggs, T. E. (2005). Feasibility and consequences of response to intervention: Examination of the issues and scientific evidence as a model for the identification of individuals with learning disabilities. *Journal of Learning Disabilities, 38*(6), 525–531.

McLoughlin, C., Zhou, Z., & Clark, E. (2005). Reflections on the development and status of contemporary special education services in China. *Psychology in the Schools, 42*(3), 325–333.

Mellard, D. F., Deshler, D. D., & Barth, A. (2004). LD identification: It's not simply a matter of building a better mousetrap. *Learning Disability Quarterly, 27*(4), 229–242.

Meng, H., Smith, S. D., Hager, K., Held, M., Liu, J., Olson, R. K., et al. (2005). DCDC2 is associated with reading disability and modulates neuronal development in the brain. *Proceedings of the National Academy of Sciences of the United States of America, 102*(47), 17053–17058.

Mintz, S. (2004). *Huck's raft: A history of American childhood.* Cambridge, MA: Harvard University Press.

Mody, M., Studdert-Kennedy, M., & Brady, S. (1997). Speech perception deficits in poor readers: Auditory processing or phonological coding? *Journal of Experimental Child Psychology, 64*(2), 199–231.

Molfese, D. L. (2000). Predicting dyslexia at 8 years of age using neonatal brain responses. *Brain and Language, 72*(3), 238–245.

Molfese, D. L., & Betz, J. C. (1988). Electrophysiological indices of the early development of lateralization for language and cognition, and their implications for predicting later development. In D. L. Molfese & S. J. Segalowitz (Eds.), *Brain lateralization in children: Developmental implications* (pp. 171–190). New York: Guilford Press.

Molfese, D. L., & Molfese, V. J. (1997). Discrimination of language skills at five years of age using event-related potentials recorded at birth. *Developmental Neuropsychology, 13*(2), 135–156.

Moores, E., Nicolson, R. I., & Fawcett, A. J. (2003). Attention deficits in dyslexia: Evidence for an automatisation deficit? *European Journal of Cognitive Psychology, 15*(3), 321–348.

Morgan, A. E., Singer-Harris, N., Bernstein, J. H., & Waber, D. P. (2000). Characteristics of children referred for evaluation of school difficulties who have adequate academic achievement scores. *Journal of Learning Disabilities, 33*(5), 489–500.

Morris, R. D., Stuebing, K. K., Fletcher, J. M., Shaywitz, S. E., Lyon, G., Shankweiler, D. P., et al. (1998). Subtypes of reading disability: Variability around a phonological core. *Journal of Educational Psychology, 90*(3), 347–373.

Morrison, G. M., & Cosden, M. A. (1997). Risk, resilience, and adjustment of individuals with learning disabilities. *Learning Disability Quarterly, 20*(1), 43–60.

Nicolson, R. I., & Fawcett, A. J. (1990). Automaticity: A new framework for dyslexia research? *Cognition, 35*(2), 159–182.

Nicolson, R. I., Fawcett, A. J., & Dean, P. (2001). Developmental dyslexia: The cerebellar deficit hypothesis. *Trends in Neurosciences, 24*(9), 508–511.

Nilles, J. M. (1999). *Electronic commerce and new ways of working: Penetration, practice and future development around the world* (Report to the Electronic Commerce and Telework Trends Project of the European Commission). Los Angeles: JALA International.

Nissen, M. J., & Bullemer, P. (1987). Attentional requirements of learning: Evidence from performance measures. *Cognitive Psychology, 19*, 1–32.

Nottebohm, F. (1971). Neural lateralization of vocal control in a passerine bird: I. Song. *Journal of Experimental Zoology, 177*(2), 229–261.

Nottebohm, F. (2005). The neural basis of birdsong. *PloS Biology, 3*(5), e164–e164.

OECD. (2000). *Literacy in the information age.* Paris: OECD Information Service.

Oliver, A., Johnson, M. H., Karmiloff-Smith, A., & Pennington, B. (2000). Deviations in the emergence of representations: A neuroconstructivist framework for analysing. *Developmental Science, 3*(1), 1.

Olofsson, H., & Servedio, M. R. (2008). Sympatry affects the evolution of genetic versus cultural determination of song. *Behavioral Ecology, 19*(3), 594–604.

Oswald, D., Coutinho, M., & Best, A. (2002). Community and school predictors of overrepresentation of minority children in special education. In D. Losen & G. Orfield (Eds.), *Racial inequity in special education* (pp. 1–14). Cambridge, MA: Harvard Education Press.

Palomo, R., Belinchon, M., & Ozonoff, S. (2006). Autism and family home movies: A comprehensive review. *Journal of Developmental and Behavioral Pediatrics, 27*, S59–S68.

Paracchini, S., Steer, C. D., Buckingham, L. L., Morris, A. P., Ring, S., Scerri, T., et al. (2008). Association of the *KIAA0319* dyslexia susceptibility gene with reading skills in the general population. *American Journal of Psychiatry, 165*(12), 1576–1584.

Paracchini, S., Thomas, A., Castro, S., Lai, C., Paramasivam, M., Wang, Y., et al. (2006). The chromosome 6p22 haplotype associated with dyslexia reduces the expression of *KIAA0319*, a novel gene involved in neuronal migration. *Human Molecular Genetics, 15*(10), 1659–1666.

Paulesu, E., Demonet, J. F., Fazio, F., McCrory, E., Chanoine, V., Brunswick, N., et al. (2001). Dyslexia: Cultural diversity and biological unity. *Science, 291*, 2165.

Paulesu, E., Frith, U., Snowling, M., Gallagher, A., Morton, J., Frackowiak,

R. S., et al. (1996). Is developmental dyslexia a disconnection syndrome?: Evidence from PET scanning. *Brain, 119*(Pt. 1), 143–157.

Peters, J. M., Waber, D. P., McAnulty, G. B., & Duffy, F. H. (2003). Event-related correlations in learning impaired children during a hybrid go/no-go choice reaction visual–motor task. *Clinical Electroencephalography, 34*, 99–109.

Piaget, J. (1963). *The origins of intelligence in children.* New York: Norton.

Pincus, J., & Tucker, G. (1985). *Behavioral neurology.* New York: Oxford University Press.

Plomin, R., & Kovas, Y. (2005). Generalist genes and learning disabilities. *Psychological Bulletin, 131*(4), 592–617.

Pringle-Morgan, W. (1896). A case of congenital word blindness. *British Medical Journal, 2*, 178.

Puolakanaho, A., Ahonen, T., Aro, M., Eklund, K., Leppannen, P. H. T., Poikkeus, A.-M., et al. (2007). Very early phonological and language skills: Estimating individual risk of reading disability. *Journal of Child Psychology and Psychiatry, and Allied Disciplines, 48*(9), 923–931.

Rabin, M., Wen, X. L., Hepburn, M., Lubs, H. A., Feldman, E., & Duara, R. (1993). Suggestive linkage of developmental dyslexia to chromosome 1p34–p36. *Lancet, 342*, 178.

Ramsey, N. F., Jansma, J. M., Jager, G., Van Raalten, T., & Kahn, R. S. (2004). Neurophysiological factors in human information processing capacity. *Brain, 127*(Pt. 3), 517–525.

Raskind, M. H., Goldberg, R. J., Higgins, E. L., & Herman, K. L. (1999). Patterns of change and predictors of success in individuals with learning disabilities: Results. *Learning Disabilities Research and Practice, 14*(1), 35.

Rumsey, J. M., Andreason, P., Zametkin, A. J., Aquino, T., King, A. C., Hamburger, S. D., et al. (1992). Failure to activate the left temporoparietal cortex in dyslexia: An oxygen 15 positron emission tomographic study. *Archives of Neurology, 49*(5), 527–534.

Rumsey, J. M., Donohue, B. C., Brady, D. R., Nace, K., Giedd, J. N., & Andreason, P. (1997). A magnetic resonance imaging study of planum temporale asymmetry in men with developmental dyslexia. *Archives of Neurology, 54*(12), 1481–1489.

Rutter, M., Graham, P. J., & Yule, W. (1970). *A neuropsychiatric study in childhood.* Philadelphia: Lippincott.

Rutter, M., & Yule, W. (1975). The concept of specific reading retardation. *Journal of Child Psychology and Psychiatry and Allied Disciplines, 16*(3), 181–197.

Rypma, B., Berger, J. S., Prabhakaran, V., Bly, B. M., Kimberg, D. Y., Biswal, B. B., et al. (2006). Neural correlates of cognitive efficiency. *NeuroImage, 33*(3), 969–979.

Sasaki, A., Sotnikova, T. D., Gainetdinov, R. R., & Jarvis, E. D. (2006). Social context-dependent singing-regulated dopamine. *Journal of Neuroscience, 26*(35), 9010–9014.

Scarborough, H. S. (1990). Very early language deficits in dyslexic children. *Child Development, 61*(6), 1728–1743.

Schneider, W., & Fisk, A. (1982a). Concurrent automatic and visual search: Can controlled processing occur without resource cost? *Journal of Experimental Psychology: General, 8*, 261–278.

Schneider, W., & Fisk, A. (1982b). Degree of consistent training: Improvements in search performance and automatic process development. *Perception and Psychophysics, 31*, 160–168.

Schneider, W., & Shiffrin, R. (1977). Controlled and automatic human information processing: I. Detection, search, and attention. *Psychological Reviews, 84*, 1–66.

Schulte-Körne, G., Grimm, T., Nöthen, M. M., Müller-Myhsok, B., Cichon, S., Vogt, I. R., et al. (1998). Evidence for linkage of spelling disability to chromosome 15. *American Journal of Human Genetics, 63*(1), 279–282.

Schumacher, J., Anthoni, H., Dahdouh, F., König, I. R., Hillmer, A. M., Kluck, N., et al. (2006). Strong genetic evidence of *DCDC2* as a susceptibility gene for dyslexia. *American Journal of Human Genetics, 78*(1), 52–62.

Scientific Learning Corporation. (2005). Improved early reading skills by students in the Springfield City School District who used Fast ForWord® to Reading 1. *MAPS for Learning: Educator Reports, 9*(25), 1–5.

Seastrom, M., Hoffman, L., Chapman, C., & Stillwell, R. (2005). *The averaged freshman graduation rate for public high schools from the common core of data school years 2001–02 and 2002–03*. Washington, DC: National Center for Education Statistics.

Senf, G. (1987). Learning disabilities as sociologic sponge: Wiping up life's spills. In S. Vaughan & C. Bos (Eds.), *Research in learning disabilities: Issues and future directions* (pp. 87–96). Boston: College Hill.

Shaywitz, B. A., Fletcher, J. M., Holahan, J. M., & Shaywitz, S. E. (1992). Discrepancy compared to low achievement definitions of reading disability: Results from the Connecticut Longitudinal Study. *Journal of Learning Disabilities, 25*(10), 639–648.

Shaywitz, B. A., Shaywitz, S. E., Blachman, B. A., Pugh, K. R., Fulbright, R. K., Skudlarski, P., et al. (2004). Development of left occipitotemporal systems for skilled reading in children after a phonologically-based intervention. *Biological Psychiatry, 55*(9), 926–933.

Shaywitz, B. A., Shaywitz, S. E., Pugh, K. R., Mencl, W. E., Fulbright, R. K., Skudlarski, P., et al. (2002). Disruption of posterior brain systems for reading in children with developmental dyslexia. *Biological Psychiatry, 52*(2), 101–110.

Shaywitz, S. E., & Shaywitz, B. A. (2005). Dyslexia (specific reading disability). *Biological Psychiatry, 57*(11), 1301–1309.

Shaywitz, S. E., & Shaywitz, B. A. (2008). Paying attention to reading: The neurobiology of reading and dyslexia. *Development and Psychopathology, 20*(4), 1329–1349.

Shaywitz, S. E., Shaywitz, B. A., Pugh, K. R., Fulbright, R. K., Constable, R. T., Mencl, W. E., et al. (1998). Functional disruption in the organization of the brain for reading in dyslexia. *Proceedings of the National Academy of Sciences of the United States of America, 95*(5), 2636–2641.

Shepherd, M. J. (2001). History lessons. In A. S. Kaufman & N. L. Kaufman

(Eds.), *Specific learning disabilities and difficulties in children and adolescents: Psychological assessment and evaluation* (pp. 3–28). Cambridge, UK: Cambridge University Press.

Shiffrin, R., & Schneider, W. (1977). Controlled and automatic human information processing: II. Perceptual learning, automatic attending, and a general theory. *Psychological Reviews, 84*, 127–190.

Silani, G., Frith, U., Demonet, J. F., Fazio, F., Perani, D., Price, C., et al. (2005). Brain abnormalities underlying altered activation in dyslexia: A voxel based morphometry study. *Brain, 128*(10), 2453–2461.

Simos, P. G., Fletcher, J., Bergman, E., Breier, J., Foorman, B., Castillo, E., et al. (2002). Dyslexia-specific brain activation profile becomes normal following successful remedial training. *Neurology, 58*(8), 1203–1213.

Simos, P. G., Fletcher, J. M., Foorman, B. R., Francis, D. J., Castillo, E. M., Davis, R. N., et al. (2002). Brain activation profiles during the early stages of reading acquisition. *Journal of Child Neurology, 17*(3), 159–163.

Singer-Harris, N., Forbes, P., Weiler, M. D., Bellinger, D., & Waber, D. P. (2001). Children with adequate academic achievement scores referred for evaluation of school difficulties: Information processing deficiencies. *Developmental Neuropsychology, 20*(3), 593–603.

Smith, S. D., Kimberling, W. J., & Pennington, B. F. (1991). Screening for multiple genes influencing dyslexia. *Reading and Writing, 3*(3), 285–298.

Smith, S. D., Kimberling, W. J., Pennington, B. F., & Lubs, H. A. (1983). Specific reading disability: Identification of an inherited form through linkage analysis. *Science, 219*, 1345–1347.

Spekman, N. J., Goldberg, R. J., & Herman, K. L. (1992). Learning disabled children grow up: A search for factors related to success in the young adult years. *Learning Disabilities Research and Practice, 7*(3), 161–170.

Spreen, O. (1988). *Learning disabled children growing up: A follow-up into adulthood.* New York: Oxford University Press.

Stanberry, L. I., Richards, T. L., Berninger, V. W., Nandy, R. R., Aylward, E. H., Maravilla, K. R., et al. (2006). Low-frequency signal changes reflect differences in functional connectivity between good readers and dyslexics during continuous phoneme mapping. *Magnetic Resonance Imaging, 24*(3), 217–229.

Stanovich, K. E. (1986). Matthew effects in reading: Some consequences of individual differences in the acquisition of literacy. *Reading Research Quarterly 21*(4), 360–407.

Stanovich, K. E., & Siegel, L. S. (1994). Phenotypic performance profile of children with reading disabilities: A regression-based test of the phonological-core variable-difference model. *Journal of Educational Psychology, 86*(1), 24–53.

Stephenson, S. (1907). Six cases of congential word-blindness affecting three generations of one family. *Opthalmoscope, 5*, 482–484.

Sternberg, R. J., & Wagner, R. K. (1982). Automatization failure in learning disabilities. *Topics in Learning and Learning Disabilities, 2*(2), 1–11.

Sternberg, S. (1966). High-speed scanning in human memory. *Science, 153*, 652–654.

Swanson, H. L., Harris, K. R., & Graham, S. (Eds.). (2003). *Handbook of learning disabilities.* New York: Guilford Press.

Tallal, P. (1980). Auditory temporal perception, phonics, and reading disabilities in children. *Brain and Language, 9*(2), 182–198.

Tallal, P., Miller, S. L., Bedi, G., Byma, G., Wang, X., Nagarajan, S. S., et al. (1996). Language comprehension in language-learning impaired children improved with acoustically modified speech. *Science, 271,* 81–84.

Tallal, P., & Piercy, M. (1975). Developmental aphasia: The perception of brief vowels and extended stop consonants. *Neuropsychologia, 13*(1), 69–74.

Tiu, R. D., Jr., Thompson, L. A., & Lewis, B. A. (2003). The role of IQ in a component model of reading. *Journal of Learning Disabilities, 36*(5), 424–436.

Tronick, E., & Reck, C. (2009). Infants of depressed mothers. *Harvard Review of Psychiatry, 17*(2), 147–156.

Tzeng, S.-J. (2007). Learning disabilities in Taiwan: A case of cultural constraints on the education of students with disabilities. *Learning Disabilities Research and Practice, 22*(3), 170–175.

VanDerHeyden, A. M., Witt, J. C., & Gilbertson, D. (2007). A multi-year evaluation of the effects of a response to intervention (RTI) model on identification of children for special education. *Journal of School Psychology, 45*(2), 225–256.

van der Leij, A., & Van Daal, V. H. P. (1999). Automatization aspects of dyslexia: Speed limitations in word identification, sensitivity to increasing task demands, and orthographic compensation. *Journal of Learning Disabilities, 32*(5), 417–428.

Veenstra-VanderWeele, J., Anderson, G. M., & Cook, E. H., Jr. (2000). Pharmacogenetics and the serotonin system: Initial studies and future directions. *European Journal of Pharmacology, 410*(2–3), 165–181.

Velayos-Baeza, A., Toma, C., Paracchini, S., & Monaco, A. P. (2008). The dyslexia-associated gene *KIAA0319* encodes highly N- and O-glycosylated plasma membrane and secreted isoforms. *Human Molecular Genetics, 17*(6), 859–871.

Verhaeghen, P., & Salthouse, T. A. (1997). Meta-analyses of age–cognition relations in adulthood: Estimates of linear and nonlinear age effects and structural models. *Psychological Bulletin, 122*(3), 231–249.

Viholainen, H., Ahonen, T., Cantell, M., Lyytinen, P., & Lyytinen, H. (2002). Development of early motor skills and language in children at risk for familial dyslexia. *Developmental Medicine and Child Neurology, 44*(11), 761–769.

Viholainen, H., Ahonen, T., Lyytinen, P., Cantell, M., Tolvanen, A., & Lyytinen, H. (2006). Early motor development and later language and reading skills in children at risk of familial dyslexia. *Developmental Medicine and Child Neurology, 48*(5), 367–373.

Waber, D. P. (1989). Rate and state: A critique of models guiding the assessment of learning disordered children. In P. R. Zelazo & R. G. Barr (Eds.), *Challenges to developmental paradigms: Implications for theory, assessment, and treatment* (pp. 29–42). Hillsdale, NJ: Erlbaum.

Waber, D. P., & Bernstein, J. H. (1995). Performance of learning-disabled and non-learning-disabled children on the Rey–Osterrieth Complex Figure (ROCF): Validation of the developmental scoring system. *Developmental Neuropsychology, 11*(2), 237–252.

Waber, D. P., Forbes, P. W., Wolff, P. H., & Weiler, M. D. (2004). Neurodevelopmental characteristics of children with learning impairments classified according to the double-deficit hypothesis. *Journal of Learning Disabilities, 37*(5), 451–461.

Waber, D. P., Isquith, P. K., Kahn, C. M., Romero, I., Sallan, S. E., & Tarbeil, N. J. (1994). Metacognitive factors in the visuospatial skills of long-term survivors of acute lymphoblastic leukemia: An experimental approach to the Rey–Osterrieth Complex Figure Test. *Developmental Neuropsychology, 10*(4), 349–367.

Waber, D. P., Marcus, D. J., Forbes, P. W., Bellinger, D. C., Weiler, M. D., Sorensen, L. G., et al. (2003). Motor sequence learning and reading ability: Is poor reading associated with sequencing deficits? *Journal of Experimental Child Psychology, 84*(4), 338–354.

Waber, D. P., Weiler, M. D., Bellinger, D. C., Marcus, D. J., Forbes, P. W., Wypij, D., et al. (2000). Diminished motor timing control in children referred for diagnosis of learning problems. *Developmental Neuropsychology, 17*(2), 181–197.

Waber, D. P., Weiler, M. D., Forbes, P. W., Bernstein, J. H., Bellinger, D. C., & Rappaport, L. (2003). Neurobehavioral factors associated with referral for learning problems in a community sample: Evidence for an adaptational model for learning disorders. *Journal of Learning Disabilities, 36*(5), 467–483.

Waber, D. P., Wolff, P. H., Forbes, P. W., & Weiler, M. D. (2000). Rapid automatized naming in children referred for evaluation of heterogeneous learning problems: How specific are naming speed deficits to reading disability? *Child Neuropsychology, 6*(4), 251–261.

Wallman, J. (1979). A minimal visual restriction experiment: Preventing chicks from seeing their feet affects later responses to mealworms. *Developmental Psychobiology, 12*(4), 391–397.

Wechsler, D. (2003). *Wechsler Intelligence Scale for Children—Fourth Edition.* New York: Psychological Corporation.

Weiler, M. D., Bernstein, J. H., Bellinger, D. C., & Waber, D. P. (2000). Processing speed in children with attention deficit/hyperactivity disorder, inattentive type. *Child Neuropsychology, 6*(3), 218–234.

Weiler, M. D., Bernstein, J., Bellinger, D., & Waber, D. P. (2002). Information processing deficits in children with attention-deficit/hyperactivity disorder, inattentive type, and children with reading disability. *Journal of Learning Disabilities, 35*(5), 448–461.

Wiler, M. D., Harris, N. S., Marcus, D. J., Bellinger, D., Kosslyn, S. M., & Waber, D. P. (2000). Speed of information processing in children referred for learning problems: Performance on a visual filtering test. *Journal of Learning Disabilities, 33*(6), 538–550.

Werner, E. E. (1993). Risk and resilience in individuals with learning disabilities: Lessons learned from the Kauai Longitudinal Study. *Learning Disabilities Research and Practice, 8*(1), 28–34.

Werner, E. E., & Smith, R. S. (1992). *Overcoming the odds: High risk children from birth to adulthood.* Ithaca, NY: Cornell University Press.

Werner, E. E., & Smith, R. S. (2001). *Journeys from childhood to midlife: Risk, resilience, and recovery.* Ithaca, NY: Cornell University Press.

Willcutt, E. G., Pennington, B. F., Olson, R. K., Chhabildas, N., & Hulslander, J. (2005). Neuropsychological analyses of comorbidity between reading disability and attention deficit hyperactivity disorder: In search of the common deficit. *Developmental Neuropsychology, 27*(1), 35–78.

Wolf, M., & Bowers, P. G. (1999). The double-deficit hypothesis for the developmental dyslexias. *Journal of Educational Psychology, 91*(3), 415–438.

Wolff, P. H., Michel, G. F., Ovrut, M., & Drake, C. (1990). Rate and timing precision of motor coordination in developmental dyslexia. *Developmental Psychology, 26,* 349–359.

Yap, R. L., & van der Leij, A. (1994). Testing the automatization deficit hypothesis of dyslexia via a dual-task paradigm. *Journal of Learning Disabilities, 27*(10), 660–665.

Zaehle, T., Wustenberg, T., Meyer, M., & Jancke, L. (2004). Evidence for rapid auditory perception as the foundation of speech processing: A sparse temporal sampling fMRI study. *European Journal of Neuroscience, 20*(9), 2447–2456.

Index

Page numbers in *italics* indicate a figure or table